The AGE REVOLUTION

The AGE REVOLUTION

Dr Charles Clark and
Maureen Clark

Vermilion
LONDON

1 3 5 7 9 10 8 6 4 2

Published in 2011 by Vermilion, an imprint of Ebury Publishing
Ebury Publishing is a Random House Group company

The Random House Group Limited Reg. No. 954009
Addresses for companies within the Random House Group can be found at
www.randomhouse.co.uk

A CIP catalogue record for this book is available from the British Library

The Random House Group Limited supports the Forest Stewardship Council®
(FSC®), the leading international forest certification organisation. All our titles that
are printed on Greenpeace approved FSC® certified paper carry the FSC® logo. Our
paper procurement policy can be found at www.randomhouse.co.uk/environment

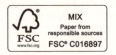

Printed and bound in Great Britain by CPI Mackays, Chatham, ME5 8TD

ISBN 9780091935474

To buy books by your favourite authors and register for offers, visit
www.randomhouse.co.uk

The information in this book has been compiled by way of general guidance in relation to the specific subjects addressed, but is not a substitute
and not to be relied on for medical, healthcare, pharmaceutical or other
professional advice on specific circumstances and in specific locations.
Please consult your GP before changing, stopping or starting any medical
treatment. So far as the author is aware the information given is correct
and up to date as at February 2011. Practice, laws and regulations all
change, and the reader should obtain up-to-date professional advice on
any such issues. The author and publishers disclaim, as far as the law
allows, any liability arising directly or indirectly from the use, or misuse, of
the information contained in this book.

All illustrations copyright © Graham Gilhooley, Zero7zero4, except on the
following pages: 97, 101, 102 (top), 103, 105, 106 (top), 107, 108 (top), 109, 115,
117, 118 (top), 119, 122 (top), 123, 125, 126 (top), 128 (top), 129, 130 (top), 133,
134 (top), 135, 136 (top), 137 © iStockphoto

Contents

Acknowledgements

WE WOULD LIKE to thank Margaret Wand, a Clinical Psychologist, for the excellent chapter on Life Changes, which incorporates a sensible and practical approach to the many situations which we encounter in later life and for which we are ill-prepared; Gill Haimes from Neal's Yard for her advice on alternative remedies, summarised in Appendix 2; and Dr David Reilly, Consultant Physician and Clinical Director of the Centre for Integrated Health at Gartnavel Hospital, for an illuminating insight into the approach to preventive health via lifestyle change.

As always, we thank our children, David and Heather, for their 'constructive' comments. Since the first book in the series was published nine years ago, the term 'children' is hardly appropriate; however, while there have been many other changes, their criticism – and critical acclaim – of their parents' efforts have remained steadfast – and honest.

Foreword

By Lucia van der Post

THE FIRST (ENCOURAGING) thing to remember about ageing is that it is so much better than the alternative. And the second thing to be said is that much of the world seems to be pre-occupied with staying young but, take it from me, growing older – with certain key provisos – has a great deal to be said for it. Nobody ever told me that when I was young.

First off growing older is really awfully interesting. There is the abiding drama of seeing lives unfold, history playing itself out, the deep pleasure of watching potential fulfilled and – the other side of the coin – the deep sadness of witnessing tragedy unfurl. Then, if one's been lucky, there's the calm that comes with knowing that certain things are settled – the family, the house, the career – and that even if we haven't had the glorious successes we might have dreamed of in our youth we have somehow come to terms with the life one has made. But the great provisos are of course: a degree of financial stability, friendship, love and companionship and, above all, health. Without health, growing older is a burdensome affair – not just for oneself but also for others. This is where the Clarks come in. I know from personal experience what Dr. Charles Clark can do on the nutritional front. His simple yet direct advice can lower insulin levels, stop arteries from clogging up, keep blindness (in diabetics) at bay, keep muscles toned and joints flexible.

Here he and his wife have joined together to provide a manual, if you like, on how to enjoy what many of us are rapidly coming to realise can be one of the best times of one's life. These days, when so much more is known about the process of ageing and, more importantly, about the essential roots of good health, there is so much we can do to help ourselves. Yes, it requires a modicum of self-discipline but most of all one needs information. With this book in hand, coupled with an open heart and a curious mind, growing older can be a life-enhancing affair, a journey not to be missed but to be enjoyed all along the way.

Introduction

OVER THE PAST nine years, we have published several books on healthy lifestyle, However, in some ways this is the most difficult book we have written; ageing is as inevitable as the changing of the seasons and no one can hold back time! But the secret is to separate the march of time from the inevitability of ageing, because although you will inevitably grow older you don't need to grow old! Most of the processes of ageing are actually a result of the way we live and are not inevitable. Most of the dreadful conditions associated with ageing – such as heart attacks, strokes and diabetes – are determined more by our lifestyle than by age. Age is merely the by-product associated with these conditions; in other words, the longer you live a life promoting these diseases, the more chance you have of developing them. The problem is knowing which advice to follow as there are so many conflicting opinions – mostly unsubstantiated and wrong! In fact, not only wrong, but almost guaranteed to accelerate the ageing process. This book is different. It will provide medically proven techniques which work!

So in many regards this is actually the easiest book we have written because most of the processes by which the 'diseases' of ageing develop are preventable or reversible. You can seriously slow or actually reverse the ageing process by following the techniques in this book, developed over many years in clinical practice. Not by following a grinding regime of exercise associated with an Olympic weight-lifter or the dietary programme of a catwalk model, but rather a simple, easily followed series of guidelines which can be achieved by everyone of any age – however advanced. And it is important to remember that *you can always make a difference, irrespective of age*. You can always make some improvement.

I have always emphasised to my patients that growing old is not a disease and ageing is not a diagnosis. There is a medical reason for everything and age is not a medical reason. So it is important to understand that the reasons for your symptoms are not 'age', or the 'march of time' or any of the other stupid reasons which I have heard some patients given by (it is to be hoped) a very small number of medical practitioners, but rather they are the result of specific medical conditions, most of which can be improved very significantly by simple, inexpensive techniques in lifestyle management.

Of course, no preventative programme will prevent all disease or replace all medication. However, by following simple guidelines you can programme your body to work for you rather than against you, and thereby slow the process of ageing, improve existing medical conditions and reduce the need for medication in many cases.

Let's begin!

1 What is ageing?

EVERYONE TALKS ABOUT ageing but what is it? Why do we experience the symptoms of creaky joints, increasing paunch, less energy and generally slowing down? More importantly, do we need to experience this? Of course, no one in his senses would attempt to arrest the progress of time, but you can slow the *effects* of time by a series of very simple, inexpensive, well-proved strategies. Because many of these symptoms are the result of the *way we live* rather than the inevitable effects of ageing.

Age is just a number. It is the way you feel and the way you look that determine your quality of life. It is often quoted that 60 is the new 40, which is probably true in terms of lifestyle. That is easy to say but it needs to be backed up by facts – and that is exactly what this book intends to achieve! Staying younger, in every sense of the word except age, involves an integrated approach involving both physical and mental health. One without the other is ineffective; as you will see, you cannot achieve a truly healthy body without a healthy mind.

Of course, this process involves the old stalwarts of diet and exercise, but although the concepts may be old, the applications are entirely new. The old concepts of diet and exercise have been shown to be ineffective in over 95% of cases but that does not mean that the concepts are wrong; on the contrary, the concepts are correct but the current forms of *application* are ineffective because they are based on completely incorrect principles, as you will see. There is no point expecting someone of 50 to follow an exercise programme designed for someone of 25 – and the weight-training regime is not very effective for maintaining cardiovascular health anyway! You need a completely dedicated health programme for *your* specific require-ments; to achieve this, the book is subdivided into the main categories of medical problems. Following the advice in all of the chapters will provide the greatest benefit, but you may wish to start with your own specific problem and drift over to the others later. Of course, many problems are present simultaneously (such as weight problems, high cholesterol and high blood pressure); this programme provides an integrated approach which addresses all of these problems at the same time.

To follow a programme to slow the ageing process, you should understand the underlying causes of ageing, but you don't need to! If you would prefer just to get on with the programme, skip to page 92 for the fundamentals.

Essentially every aspect of you comes from only two sources, either

▪ **in your genes, meaning you were born programmed to be that way, or**

▪ **acquired, which means you developed that way because of your lifestyle.**

Now we are all accustomed to reading in the media about how important your genes are, especially as the causes of particular diseases, but actually this is complete nonsense in the majority of cases. Genes cause only a very small proportion of individuals to develop diseases and have little effect on ageing in most cases. Of course, all disease patterns are different and it is impossible to generalise, but by far the majority of cases of heart disease, diabetes, strokes, obesity, raised cholesterol, hypertension and arthritis develop as a direct result of our lifestyle. So if you adopt the correct lifestyle, you may not completely eradicate these conditions but you will certainly reduce their effects considerably and can significantly reduce the likelihood of their developing in the first place.

That is quite a statement!

By simply changing your pattern of life – not much, just a little – you can prevent the unpleasant effects of these diseases in many cases. Before explaining how to achieve this minor miracle you need to know the basics of how the body ages to understand how to slow the process from 'fast forward' to 'pause', or even 'rewind'!

As you know, the body is made up of lots of tiny cells, about 50 trillion (that's 50,000,000,000,000) in total and that is definitely a lot of zeros! The powerhouse of our bodies lies in each of these cells which use the energy and oxygen delivered by the bloodstream to power the cells. The cells act in unison as specific organs (such as the liver, the heart, the brain and the muscles) and enable all of the myriad of bodily functions to occur. Obviously such a complex machine as the body has the capacity to age and this occurs when the cells become less efficient and waste products build up in the cell until it finally dies. The secret is to provide the cells with the building blocks they need to survive and to clear away the cellular waste before it accumulates.

Nutrition is actually at the basis of everything we do and everything we are. And yet it is something that we hardly ever think about! The well-known expression 'You are what you eat' is actually more true than you realise. Our bodies have an incredible capacity for withstanding gross nutritional abuses for many years, without apparent disturbance, but in actual fact you are simply storing up problems for the future when this happens. And actually, what is more relevant is the fact that this does not need to be the case. To enjoy excellent food, excellent nutrition and immeasurable health advantages is relatively simple, relatively inexpensive and relatively quick!

Nutritional Coherence is the term we use for incorporating nutrition into every aspect of our lifestyle, because it is the basis of most of our lifestyle. No one would argue the fact that health is at the heart – literally – of our quality of life. However, few understand that what we eat is the single most important part of that quality. Of course, there are many other stresses on the system, such as concerns over occupation, family, personal health, etc. But actually most of these concerns can be alleviated to a very large degree by maintaining an adequate level of nutrition, which means a high level of antioxidants (preventing the formation of free radicals which cause many diseases) and maintenance of a stable blood sugar which enables balanced concentration and mood.

Health is a very difficult measure to quantify simply because we always consider health to be a 'right' – until it is taken from us! Therefore we tend to quantify 'ill health' rather than 'health'. When we become sick we consider that we are unwell. But actually, the sensible approach to the situation should be to approach it as a 'wellness' situation which has developed into an 'unwell' situation. In other words, we must adopt the principle of prevention rather than cure. And the point about prevention is all it requires is some aspect of positive intervention to prevent the inevitable consequences. The majority of diseases of modern living are preventable, and are caused by poor lifestyle. Diabetes, heart disease, obesity and arthritis are all the consequences, to a large degree, of our lifestyle. They are not inevitable. In relatively small numbers of cases, there is a genetic component, but I would stress that this is relatively small.

So in other words what we are saying is that you can actually change the future by replacing the old (inevitable) with the probable. And it is, on the balance of probability, very likely that you will not develop heart disease or diabetes or stroke or obesity simply by making a number of lifestyle changes. Of course, it is impossible to prevent all of these diseases in every individual, but most conditions are preventable simply because they are due to lifestyle changes, and we can reverse the change.

Nutritional Coherence essentially involves making nutrition a coherent part of lifestyle, and integrating nutrition into other aspects of lifestyle.

This involves a complete change in the approach to your lifestyle. It does not involve time or expense but rather a rethinking of the way you live your life. In simple terms, it means putting you and your family first! While this may seem relatively straightforward and simple, and perhaps selfish to some minds, it really is not. If you place your health at the front of your priorities, you will have a much, much higher standard of living and enjoyment of life.

What does this mean? Actually, it means really simple changes to your lifestyle which will have an incredibly disproportionate effect on standard of living.

2 There is an alternative to drugs

THAT'S QUITE A statement. Does it mean we are against medication? Certainly not!

As a consultant surgeon of 30 years' standing it would be ridiculous for me to state that we do not need drugs. Drugs are an essential part of medicine and an essential part of health.

But the point is that we are not using drugs in the way in which they were intended.

Medication is an adjunct to a healthy lifestyle, not a replacement. Use common sense to prevent common ailments.

In the majority of cases, medication is used to manipulate the *effects* of the condition, whereas we need to remove the *cause* of the disease – otherwise it will simply recur.

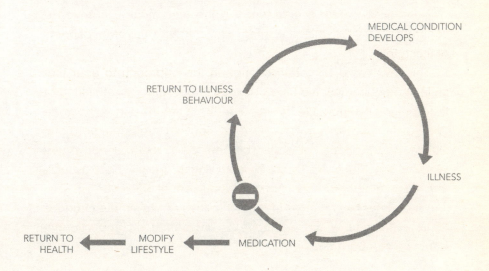

MEDICAL CONDITION DEVELOPS

RETURN TO ILLNESS BEHAVIOUR

ILLNESS

RETURN TO HEALTH ← MODIFY LIFESTYLE ← MEDICATION

Let us take some serious ailments to demonstrate the ineffectiveness of drugs in isolation without associated lifestyle changes.

It is well accepted that in heart disease, the coronary arteries become blocked, preventing the heart receiving the oxygen and nutrition it needs and therefore heart muscle dies, and if enough heart muscle dies then we die! So the underlying cause, in most but not all cases, is the blocking of the coronary arteries. This can occur, in the main, by

■ **Raised cholesterol levels in the blood blocking the artery.**

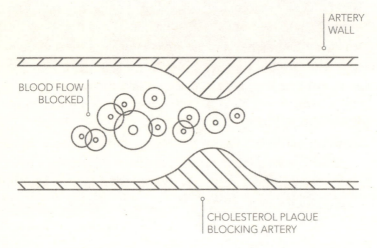

ARTERY WALL

BLOOD FLOW BLOCKED

CHOLESTEROL PLAQUE BLOCKING ARTERY

■ **Smoking causing constriction of the blood vessels and therefore blocking arteries.**

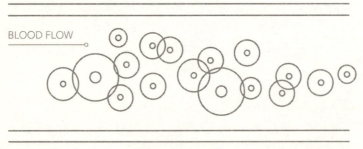

BLOOD FLOW

NORMAL ARTERY

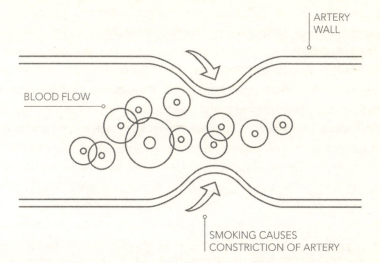

Stress causing constriction of the arteries blocking the blood flow to the heart.

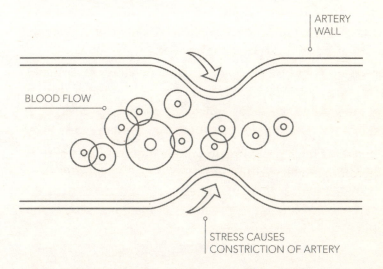

Or, in the majority of cases a combination of all three!

The treatment for such a heart condition would logically be to remove the causes of the condition and so you should remove the cause of cholesterol in the blood in the arteries, stop smoking, reduce the stress in your life.

In reality, the commonest treatment for heart conditions is prescribing drugs called statins, which reduce the level of cholesterol in the blood.

While the statins are effective in reducing cholesterol they are not effective in isolation and in fact the mortality rate in patients with statins is still extremely high.

A similar approach is taken in the management of all of the major conditions associated with ageing: diabetes, hypertension, strokes, arthritis and obesity. In all of these conditions, drugs are prescribed in the first instance, usually in place of lifestyle changes to treat the condition, and they do not work. Unless you actively change your lifestyle to combat these conditions, the chances are that you will develop one or more in your lifetime. The good news is that it is relatively simple to change your lifestyle and you can actually enjoy your life much more by doing so.

There are essentially four components to achieve success in the alternative route to drugs:

- **Changing your diet, which will reduce the risks of diabetes, heart disease and raised cholesterol.**
- **Lowering stress levels by adopting a positive attitude and in this regard it is essential to have positive adaptive strategies for the various situations which occur as we age. This will reduce the risks of many diseases by lowering stress levels naturally and has the additional advantage of developing a much greater sense of relaxation and wellbeing, which inevitably improves quality of life.**
- **Exercise, which need not be hours at the gym, but a balanced plan to improve circulation.**

Techniques to achieve this will be described in later chapters.

- **And, obviously, do not smoke. This stipulation is probably unnecessary for the majority of readers of this book, because simply by reading the book you are adopting a positive attitude towards the future and are unlikely to be smoking.**

If you want to achieve a quick fix, then simply follow the diet accurately and closely, and you will reduce the risk of diabetes, reduce your cholesterol, reduce heart disease and the chance of strokes within a relatively short period.

However, if you wish to really improve your quality of life and achieve the maximum benefit from this programme, not only reducing the risks of disease but also improving your enjoyment of life and quality of life, then really it is essential to read the chapters on positive mindset and reduction in stress.

Although obviously we are discussing a physical problem here with ageing, in actual fact most problems originate from a negative attitude of mind and a negative approach to the various strategies described.

The basis of this programme is essentially prevention and positivity. What does this mean? Let us consider the actions of medications for a moment. When you take medication, it means that you already have the problem. We are accepting that the problem exists and will not go away, and that the only way to deal with it is to take medication to control it but not to prevent it or reverse it.

For example, if you have diabetes you take medication to lower the blood sugar, but eventually this is not effective because the diet followed usually makes diabetes deteriorate, so eventually you take more medication until finally many diabetics have to inject with insulin.

So really when we take drugs we are dealing with an 'anti-problem'. Every aspect of drugs is to accept the problem and counteract its effects, *rather than dealing with the problem itself,* and that approach is doomed to failure from the outset. To reiterate, this is not to suggest that drugs are not essential – they are – but always in conjunction with a preventive approach to the problem. For example:

- **We take 'anti' depressants for depression, rather than trying to treat the cause of depression.**
- **We take 'anti' biotics for infection.**
- **We take 'anti' inflammatory drugs for arthritis.**

If you think about it for a moment all you are actually doing is relieving the symptoms. But you are not actually taking away the problem in any shape or form.

So when we take drugs, this is a negative act in that we are accepting the problem is irreversible and we are simply giving it something to control it, or if not control it, relieve some of the symptoms.

This does not mean that drugs are bad. But it does mean that it is a rather strange way of looking at the problem. Surely it would be more sensible to try to treat the cause of the condition, and remove as many of the causes as possible, and then if you are left with any symptoms afterwards to treat the residual symptoms with drugs.

So, for example, in a patient who has severe knee pain from arthritis, surely it would be more sensible for him or her to lose weight and relieve some of the strain on the joints, as a first principle, rather than just treat the pain with more and more anti-inflammatory drugs

Or in a case of a patient with heart disease and raised cholesterol, surely it would be more sensible to lower the cholesterol initially by diet, rather than just to lower it artificially by using cholesterol-lowering agents such as statins. In other words, if you adopt an alternative route to drugs, what you are actually doing is adopting a positive approach to prevention rather than a negative approach of acceptance of the condition and merely treating the symptoms. But that positive approach has to come from a positive mindset initially, a mindset that believes that 'failure is not an option' (quotation from the approach to the Apollo 13 mission). A mindset that says that you want to take control of your own body back from the symptoms and medication that it is receiving.

So you can appreciate that this is certainly not an 'anti' drug approach. On the contrary, it is a pro-drug approach but an approach which means that we only use drugs appropriately where necessary and actually take as much of the control back ourselves, which we can do by positive, preventative strategies. To understand how this can be achieved, you really need to understand where the main problems come from. It's not that difficult; most of medicine is relatively simple to understand when it is explained in a simple way. Let us take the main problems of heart disease and stroke caused by blocking of the arteries from raised cholesterol. The simplest place to begin is where the cholesterol comes from. Cholesterol comes from your food, everybody knows that.

Well, everyone may know that but in fact it is wrong! In actual fact, 85% of the cholesterol in your blood is made by your own liver and surprisingly it is made in response to sugar. So if you have eggs for breakfast, which is made up of about 20% cholesterol, this does not stimulate the liver to produce cholesterol, and your cholesterol levels will decrease.

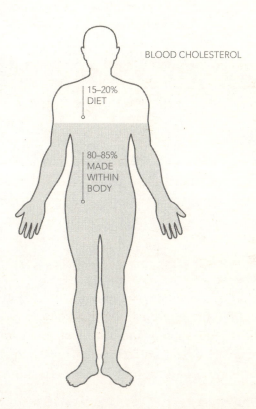

BLOOD CHOLESTEROL

15–20%
DIET

80–85%
MADE
WITHIN
BODY

If on the other hand you have something starchy for breakfast, like toast or cereal, this stimulates the liver to produce cholesterol, and cholesterol levels rise.

This seems rather odd! In fact, it is the opposite of most of the information provided by public health sources. What evidence could possibly support this eccentric opinion?

ACTUALLY IT IS ACCEPTED MEDICAL FACT IN STANDARD MEDICAL REFERENCE TEXTBOOKS. In other words, it is carbohydrates in your diet that increase blood levels of cholesterol. Established medical fact!

So if you cut out many of the starchy foods like potatoes, pasta and rice, this will prevent the blood fat levels rising in your body and if you replace it with other foods, such as egg and meat and proteins, this will cause the blood fat levels to reduce.

And if the cholesterol levels reduce, you automatically reduce the risk of heart disease and strokes and conditions such as diabetes. So simply by reducing certain sugars in your diet, you reduce the cholesterol levels and reduce your risks of these awful conditions. You also reduce the risks of conditions which result, such as obesity, hypertension and arthritis.

Obviously, if you reduce the foods that cause sugar levels to rise in your blood, then you reduce the risk of diabetes. So by simply reducing the levels of starchy foods (meaning carbohydrates and sugars) in your diet, you have automatically reduced the risk of heart disease, strokes, diabetes and arthritis.

Having made this sweeping statement, we now need to look at the foods that make up a typical diet, and the foods that you should include and how, in order to achieve this incredible improvement in health.

Essentially there are five main food groups:

- **Carbohydrates**
- **Proteins**
- **Fats**
- **Vitamins**
- **Minerals**

Of course the sixth and most important component of our diet is WATER, because if you do not take in enough water, this will undoubtedly precipitate many medical conditions, or exacerbate many existing ones.

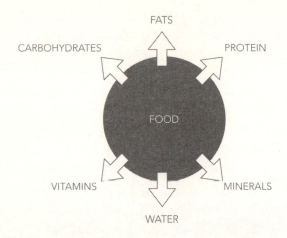

The importance is in ensuring we obtain the correct proportions of these various food groups. In summary, what they do is as follows:

Protein

Protein is essentially the building block of life. Almost all of your body is made up of protein and fats, and certainly all of the structural part of your body is protein: bones, muscles, organs, skin, hair, teeth and nails are all made up mainly of body protein.

And the only way that you can obtain protein is from a healthy diet. We cannot store protein in the body, unlike fat, and therefore you have to keep topping up the supplies of protein to make sure that your body remains healthy. By far the best supply of protein is from animal sources such as meat, fish, poultry, eggs and cheese. There is certainly protein in vegetables but to a much lesser degree. The only complete source of protein in plants is in soya products. So unless you are a vegetarian, it is essential to add a certain amount of animal protein to your diet, preferably fish or chicken.

The other important reason for increasing the amount of protein in your diet is that the immune system, which fights disease and cancer, is made up essentially of protein. And as we cannot store protein in the body, unless you provide your body with sufficient

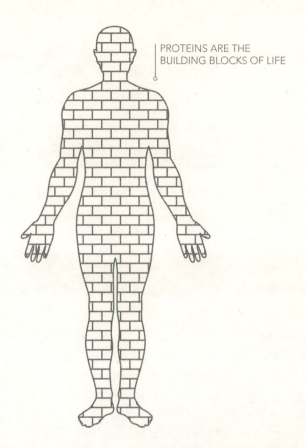

PROTEINS ARE THE
BUILDING BLOCKS OF LIFE

protein to keep fighting various problems that occur as we get older, the immune system, or the protective mechanism of the body, will be impaired and your ability to fight off infection and cancer will be reduced.

So in essence, it is absolutely essential to maintain good-quality protein in your diet. This need not be expensive. There is no difference between the quality of protein in the best fillet steak and in, for example, sardines or tinned salmon. To the body, the protein is exactly the same. When we ingest it, it is broken down to its component parts (called amino acids) in the bowel which are absorbed into the body and then re-formed into the body proteins which we have.

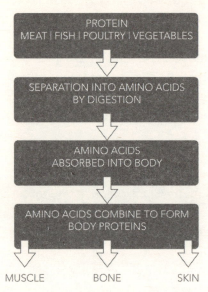

There is absolutely no difference between the protein in muscle or brain tissue in yourself or in that of a sardine! The basic building blocks are exactly the same, the only difference is we form them in a different way. But what is essential is that you take in enough of this essential food to make your body proteins which break down with age and need to be constantly replenished.

Fats

There has been a huge amount of adverse criticism regarding fats in our diet. Much of this is well justified; the trans fats which are incorporated in manufactured and processed foods such as margarine, cakes, biscuits, and many processed pies are extremely dangerous to health. These forms of fats which occur in convenience foods and ready-made foods are completely unnatural. They do not occur anywhere in nature and have been made in laboratories. As such, when they are incorporated into the body structure, they are weak and cause problems, for example blood vessels to rupture and cell walls to be much weaker, causing disease.

But this does certainly not mean that all fats are bad. On the contrary, many fats are not only good for you but absolutely essential. We have a number of essential fatty acids which you have probably heard of called omega 3 fatty acids and omega 6 fatty acids, and these are found in certain foods which we will explain later, but the most important thing is that not all fat is bad. Fat provides a significant amount of energy, and as long as the correct fats are ingested, they will certainly not make you put on weight.

So, in summary, fats which are good for you include the omega 3 fatty acids and the omega 6 fatty acids, which are found in food such as fatty fish (herring, mackerel, salmon, sardines and tuna), eggs, nuts and vegetable oils (such as flax seed). In the case of omega 6 fatty acids, these are found in eggs and seeds (particularly sunflower, safflower, grains and vegetable oils).

As you can see, all of these are extremely healthy foods and should be incorporated in your diet. Much more importantly, they are not expensive. This is not advocating some expensive and exclusive dietary programme, but rather the opposite; the application of sensible, healthy and inexpensive foods to health.

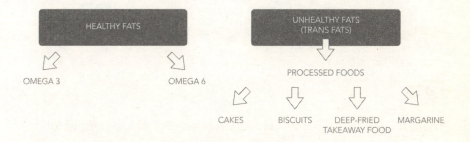

Carbohydrates

The first fact to realise is that:

CARBOHYDRATES ARE NOT ESSENTIAL FOR LIFE

I appreciate that this will seem absolute heresy when you consider all of the advice you are given but the fact is that there is no carbohydrate in nature which is essential for life. The word carbohydrate means simply 'sugar' as carbohydrates are nothing more than sugar molecules joined together.

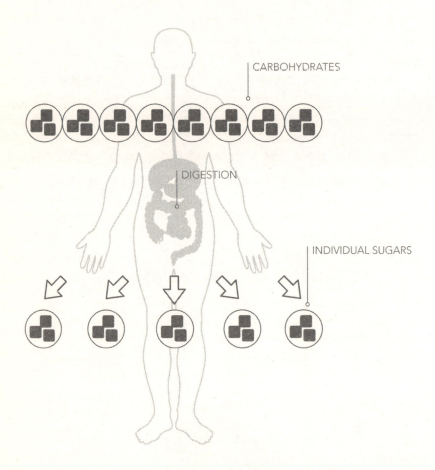

So when you eat breakfast cereal in the morning, it is essentially 75% carbohydrate, which is 75% sugar. This is not made apparent on the label, but it is a fact. So if you just imagine that the plate is full of 75% sugar (without adding sugar or anything else to your meal) that is what you are eating. Frightening isn't it?

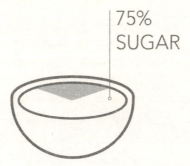

75%
SUGAR

The importance is that these refined carbohydrates provide no nutrition whatsoever. In fact, many of them are so poor in nutrition (such as certain breakfast cereals and white bread) that the government insists, by law, that vitamins and minerals are added to provide some element of nutrition.

The relevance is that, as we grow older, we need more nutrition – not less – to combat the effects of ageing. This is achieved by providing the necessary nutrition that we need in the form of protein, fats, vitamins and minerals to build up our bodies to fight the various ravages of age such as infection and cancer. This is certainly not to say that carbohydrates are bad, they most certainly are not. The worst carbohydrates are those refined carbohydrates which are found in:

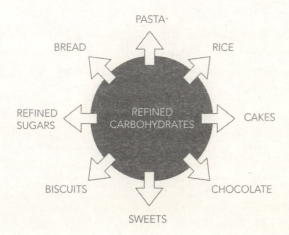

- Breakfast cereals
- Bread
- Pasta and rice
- Cakes and confectionery
- Most fruit juices (where sugar has been added)
- Beers and ciders and fortified wine such as sherry

But there are many healthy carbohydrates that are associated with all of the vitamins, minerals and proteins that we require, and these are primarily found in fresh vegetables.

So you can see that by following this diet you are not following a low carbohydrate diet, but rather a high carbohydrate diet as there is no restriction on the carbohydrates, particularly the unrefined carbohydrates, which are present in fresh vegetables. This is a Low Refined-Carbohydrate Diet.

Vitamins and minerals

It is not important to understand the exact reasons why you need vitamins and minerals but much more important to know where they come from. Essentially, vitamins and minerals are required in tiny quantities by every cell in the body for all of its reactions but the emphasis is on tiny quantities and the most important aspect is where they come from. All of the vitamins and minerals that you need, surprisingly, are present in most of the foods which you would consider healthy! In other words, the following foods include all of the essential vitamins and minerals for health.

- Meat, fish, shellfish, poultry, dairy produce and eggs
- Fruit and vegetables

And that's it!

You can see, with a diet which is incredibly varied with all of the delicious foods that you enjoy, you will include all of the

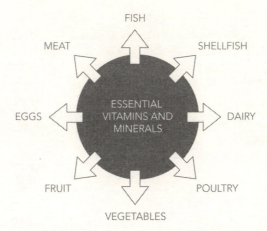

essential vitamins and minerals in your diet. And it is important to realise that many of the vitamins are actually fat soluble, which means that they can only be absorbed if they are contained in fat, such as vitamins A, D, E and K. So unless you include fats in your diet you cannot absorb these vitamins and therefore you will become ill.

But, just as the foods which contain these essential vitamins and minerals are important, of equal importance is to emphasise the foods which contain very little of these essential nutrients. Most cereals and most processed foods and many pre-prepared foods contain very little nutrition in the form of vitamins and minerals. You cannot obtain many of the vitamins essential for life unless you consume a diet which includes fresh vegetables.

Without vitamins and minerals, it does not matter how well you think you are eating; you will undoubtedly become ill because the building blocks of life will not be present.

But why do we need these vitamins and minerals and what do they actually do? Well, the real problem with ageing is something called free radical formation. Free radicals are molecules which have lost an electron and so they have to grab an electron from another molecule nearby.

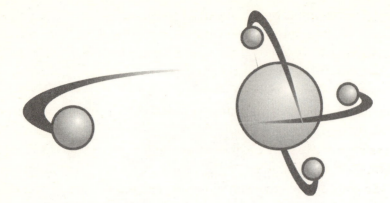

This sets off a cascade of reactions within the body which destabilises all of these 50 trillion cells and gradually damages each of the cells and slowly ages us by increasing the ratio of damaged cells to good cells. It is obviously not important for you to understand anything about free radical formation but it is important to understand how you can stop it happening because that is one of the main techniques to slow the ageing process. If you provide these cells with an extra electron, then they stop bumping into each other and damaging one another and slow the damage of cells to the body.

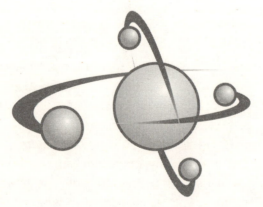

And the way that this is achieved is by eating foods which contain 'antioxidants', which provide the extra electron to free radicals, thus preventing the free radical from causing any damage to the body. Antioxidants are a subject of the media all the time and they sound very complex indeed but actually they are very simple. Essentially, if you enjoy a diet which has a high proportion of fresh vegetables, they will contain all of the antioxidants that you need. The main antioxidants are vitamins A, C and E, so a diet high in vegetables such as 'coloured vegetables', peppers and carrots and avocados, will include all of the antioxidants you could possibly need to wipe out these free radicals AND SLOW THE AGEING PROCESS CONSIDERABLY.

So you can see that, with some very simple changes to your diet, you can slow the ageing process at the cellular level, and that is the process which contributes to general ageing. A simple technique with a huge effect on the quality of life.

And the single most important determinant of ageing is:

> **SUGAR!**

How can this be? How can sugar, the simple white substance that sweetens our food, be the single most important cause of ageing?

Because sugar molecules infiltrate themselves into the body proteins and weaken them, causing proteins that make up the structure of our bodies to crack and split.

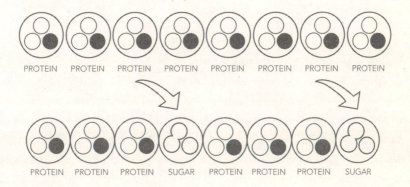

Obviously, when we talk about damage to structural proteins, that does not mean anything to the ordinary individual, but when you talk about wrinkling of the skin and hardening of the arteries and heart disease and stiffening of the joints causing arthritis, that makes much more sense. And these are exactly the effects that sugar has on our body proteins.

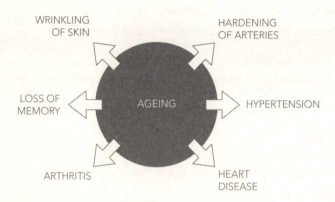

EFFECTS OF
AGEING

WRINKLING
OF SKIN

HARDENING
OF ARTERIES

LOSS OF
MEMORY

AGEING

HYPERTENSION

ARTHRITIS

HEART
DISEASE

However, if ageing of the skin and hardening of the arteries and stiffening of the joints are not enough, sugar has even worse effects on our body! All of the processes which occur within these millions and trillions of individual cells are controlled by proteins, and if sugar infiltrates the protein and causes it to be damaged, then the reactions within these cells become slow and we age and slowly die. Yes, that's right, sugars contribute towards the ageing process.

Not only does sugar affect the workings within each cell to slow it down and gradually slow us down, but sugars break down the proteins that act as antioxidants in the body protecting us against these 'free radicals' which we mentioned earlier which are also part of the ageing process. So sugar is slowing down the proteins in our cells that keep us effectively normal, causing ageing, and slowing down the proteins that are antioxidants which help to protect us.

Can sugars have even more bad effects? The answer is yes. Increased sugar in your diet actually increases the cholesterol in your blood, causing heart disease and strokes. In actual fact, most of the cholesterol in your blood does not come from your diet but from your own liver and it is made there in response to sugar, indirectly via a hormone called insulin.

So you can see that increased sugar in the diet causes ageing in many different ways, by:

- Damaging the structural proteins of the body, causing ageing of the skin with wrinkles, hardening of the arteries with effects on heart attacks and strokes, and stiffening of the joints with arthritis
- Affecting the proteins in every individual cell, which slows down the cell and finally kills it, the ultimate end point of ageing
- Increasing the blood cholesterol level, which further contributes to hardening of the arteries, heart attacks and strokes.

But it is not the normal white sugar that is the main problem. We can easily cut down on white sugar intake. It is the 'hidden sugars' that cause the real problem, because you do not realise that you are eating sugar. What do we mean by 'hidden sugars'? Foods such as cereals are actually made of 75% carbohydrates, and as carbohydrates are simply sugar molecules joined together this means that they are actually 75% sugar.

So when you have your breakfast cereal in the morning, what you do not realise is that 75% of it is converted into sugar in the body, even though you do not add any sugar to it. Pasta, rice, and bread are each about 73–75% carbohydrate which means that they are converted to 75% sugar in your body. When you next look at the plate of rice before you, think of it as three-quarters sugar! Or if you have a slice of bread, think of it as three-quarters sugar; in the average slice of bread there are approximately 3–4 teaspoons of carbohydrate which means 3–4 teaspoons of sugar. A very sobering thought.

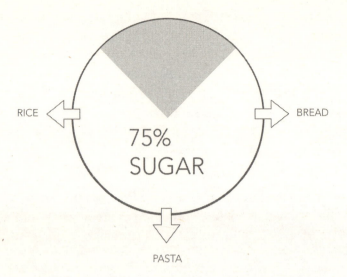

And as you can see that sugar contributes so much to the ageing process in many different ways, it would seem obvious that one of the things we need to do to combat ageing is to cut out much of the sugar in our diet, which means reducing many of the carbohydrates in our diet.

> **SO THE FIRST STEP TO SLOWING THE AGEING PROCESS IS TO EXCLUDE REFINED CARBOHYDRATES FROM YOUR DIET!**

3 Recognise the signs

THE SIGNS OF ageing would seem relatively obvious, even to a casual observer, but in actual fact they are not as obvious as you might think, because although you measure ageing by appearance on the *outside,* the really important changes are taking place *inside* the body. In essence, the changes that are occurring inside the body are *causing* the external changes. As a simple example from the previous chapter, when someone is overweight it is usually attributed to excessive overeating but the excess fat is actually caused by a medical condition of raised levels of the hormone insulin. So if you try to slim by simply eating minimal calories (or starving, as a more accurate description) this will always be unsuccessful because the underlying cause of the problem has not been addressed, i.e. the medical problem *inside* the body.

The obvious signs of ageing are those which have already occurred and which are permanent, such as wrinkling of the skin, but rather than dwelling on permanent changes, it is more important to emphasise the positive changes you can make to prevent the external signs of ageing, or if they have happened, how to prevent any further progression.

To return to the Introduction to the book, you cannot stop the process of ageing for obvious reasons. You will naturally age because that is a natural progression of time.

However, to reiterate the sentiments of the Introduction, although you will inevitably *grow* older, you don't necessarily need to age with all the ravages of time, because many of the so-called 'ravages of time' are actually caused by lifestyle and are not the result of an inevitable 'natural progression' of time.

Of course, there are some individuals who will develop serious illnesses such as cancer or heart disease irrespective of lifestyle, but the majority of effects of the ageing process *in the majority of individuals* are results of abuses in lifestyle.

For a moment, let us leave aside the obvious signs of ageing which occur in the later stages and let us examine the earliest signs of the ageing process – *a gradual slowing up of all of our bodily functions*.

The problem is that the process is so slow and gradual that we don't actually notice the warning signs until it is too late. But why should this be so? Why should our body functions deteriorate with time? We always consider this to be inevitable but, once again, although it is inevitable to *age*, it is not inevitable to *age rapidly*.

AGE IS NOT A DIAGNOSIS! There is no disease called 'ageing'. So, like any other medical condition, there must be an underlying reason for the changes associated with ageing, and, by identifying the reason(s), you can then proceed to address them.

There are many effects of ageing but one of the central causes of the entire process of the slowing up of body functions is gradual deterioration in the body's proteins and poor circulation to all of the tissues, not just the muscles, but more particularly the organs them-selves. This means, in effect, that the following symptoms occur during the ageing process which are characteristic of the problem:

1. Weakening of muscle strength. It seems inevitable as we grow older that the power in our muscles will become impaired; however, even apart from the obvious examples of taking regular exercise, you can vastly improve muscle power by many other techniques that probably you did not realise. Similarly, other effects of ageing can be improved in the same manner.
2. The slowing of the mental processes, possibly leading to Alzheimer's disease or other forms of dementia.
3. Redistribution of body fat, with a more 'apple' appearance for a man (deposition of body fat around the upper abdomen) and a more 'pear' shape appearance for a woman, with deposition of body fat on the hips, thighs and lower abdomen.

4. Generalised aches and pains in joints, with the development of arthritis.
5. Heart disease, once again leading to restriction of our physical activities.
6. Shortness of breath on exertion.

There are many other symptoms and signs of ageing but these are probably the most common. All of these symptoms and signs occur in the later stages of ageing – *but most can be addressed in the early stages of the disease process by simple and inexpensive changes in lifestyle.* So it is obviously important to realise that the single most important feature in the ageing process is a gradual slowing down of bodily functions!

Much more importantly, it is desperately important to address this problem *by making lifestyle changes before the effects on the body become permanent.*

We have seen in the previous chapter how poor diet can lead to very significant problems with the development of many diseases and you will understand in the following chapter how stress and anxiety can accelerate these problems. But why should they occur?

We have already seen that structural proteins in the body, such as those in blood vessels, bones and muscles, can become weakened by the insertion of sugar molecules into the protein chains.

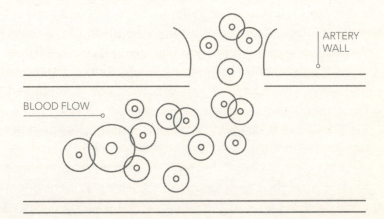

ARTERY WALL

BLOOD FLOW

SUGAR WEAKENS STRUCTURAL PROTEIN, CAUSING RUPTURE OF BLOOD VESSELS

However, what is not quite so apparent is the fact that these weaknesses do have a specific name and it is:

AGE!

No, not the ageing process that you think it is, but rather a medical process called

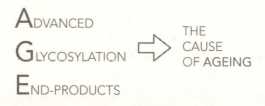

Advanced Glycosylation End-products are the effects of the weakening of body proteins by the insertion of sugar molecules, described above. In fact, the ageing process is to a very large extent contributed to by the amount of sugar that you eat. But there is obviously much more to it than this and, to obtain the maximum benefit, it is essential that you follow the programme in all of its aspects: diet, exercise, and stress relief.

Probably the most important aspect of this is *awareness*. Be aware of your own body and be aware of the signs and symptoms as they develop. By doing so you can identify problems before they fully develop, enabling physical preventative action to address these issues. Don't consider ageing as an inevitable pessimistic downward spiral, but rather as a process which occurs but to which there are effective solutions to improve the associated quality of life.

You wouldn't normally let your car run into a dangerous condition before fixing the problem, so why do this with your body? The government can ensure the safety of your vehicle with a yearly MOT; you need to perform a daily MOT on your health! You don't need the medical profession to do yearly medical checks, you can do most of the preventive maintenance yourself as most of the problems of ageing are very obvious to the patient by the symptoms that they feel!

Let's examine this major symptom of 'slowing down'. It does not seem a very strong medical diagnosis, and I am sure you won't see many doctors writing 'slowing down' on a medical certificate, but it is probably the most important symptom that we have as a warning sign for the future. Once we have developed the more obvious symptoms of pain in the chest, shortness of breath, ankle joint and knee joint pain, loss of memory ... the list is endless, the quality of life at that stage becomes very poor indeed.

There is no need to endure most of these symptoms. The number of slim individuals requiring hip replacements is insignificant compared with those who are grossly overweight. Being overweight is one of your body's main indicators that there is something wrong inside the body. Fat is controlled by the hormone insulin, which in turn is controlled by having too many sugars and carbohydrates in your diet. Body fat itself is much more dangerous because it is an indicator of potentially serious medical conditions inside the body, rather than its physical and cosmetic disadvantages. The major physical effect of body fat is to exacerbate arthritis, particularly in hip and knee joints. So if you want to alleviate the pain of arthritis in the lower limbs, reduce your body fat by appropriate dietary changes – which are not difficult!

Similarly, to reduce the ageing effects on the brain, improve the blood flow to the brain by several simple techniques:

■ Stop smoking

Smoking constricts the vessels and increases the blockage of blood vessels by cholesterol, preventing the circulation of blood to very important organs (including the brain) and therefore directly contributing to memory loss.

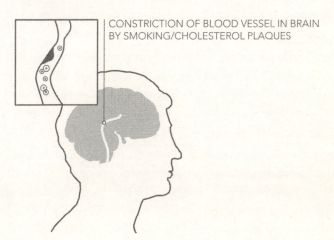

CONSTRICTION OF BLOOD VESSEL IN BRAIN BY SMOKING/CHOLESTEROL PLAQUES

Of course, you cannot prevent Alzheimer's and other dementias entirely by techniques such as diet and not smoking, but you can reduce the likelihood very significantly and, much more important, improve your quality of life immensely by this simple technique.

Heart disease

No one would argue that heart disease is primarily a result of smoking, poor diet with raised cholesterol and high blood pressure. Of course, once again, there is a proportion of the population that will develop heart disease due to genetic effects, but once again it is relatively small compared to the general prevalence of heart disease in the community.

All of these causes of heart disease are simply treated by changing lifestyle. Apart from the risk of death from heart disease, the very poor quality of life for many years associated with coronary disease, with the constant struggle to survive, is probably an even more significant reason to take all possible preventive measures.

Stress and anxiety

Recognise the effects of stress and anxiety. Ignore the symptoms of stress at your peril. The graveyards are overflowing with individuals who tried to ignore stress! And certainly don't try to simply use medication as a prop to solve the problem, *because it will not*. Medication in this particular situation serves merely to mask the problem, not to address it.

Recognise stress is happening, accept the fact, and deal with it. The way to deal with stress is explained in some detail in Chapter 4.

The most important aspect of this chapter is to make you aware of the ways in which your body changes with age. Don't consider age to be a depressing situation where the progress and the development of ageing diseases are inevitable. On the contrary, think of it as a warning process like the oil light flashing on your car; in the majority of cases you can actually do something about it. You would never consider not putting oil in your car; why leave your body in the same situation?

Spend a fraction of the time correcting your body's illnesses, as you would on polishing your car or cleaning the house, and you will prevent many of the problems from becoming 'inevitable'.

The secret of a healthy lifestyle and high standard of living in your later years lies, in the main, in your own hands. Be positive and go forward!

4 Accentuate the positive

ALTHOUGH WE HAVE concentrated on physical illnesses, a fact seldom realised is that many physical illnesses are exacerbated *or actually caused* by stress. In other words, our mental state can have immense implications for our physical health.

Stress is a major factor in many illnesses, and therefore it is absolutely essential to control stress. But what is stress?

This must be probably one of the most overused words in the English language! Everyone knows what stress is; it's when someone is agitated for some reason or other and this seems to be a normal part of life. But it is not a normal part of life and it is certainly not simple.

Before explaining the basis of 'stress' and how it can make you so very unhealthy it would be important to explain how this 'stress reaction' occurs. Because 'stress' controls virtually every action we make!

Basically we have two separate nervous systems in our bodies. The nervous system that travels down the backbone is known to everyone and this controls our conscious sensation and movement, such as walk, talk, run, smile.

But in actual fact this nervous system in the backbone accounts for only about 1% of all the actions that you do. The 99% remaining make up all the things that you don't think about but which are absolutely essential to life, such as breathing, heart rate, circulation, digestion, and all of the chemical reactions that occur in the 50 trillion cells of your body every fraction of a second of every

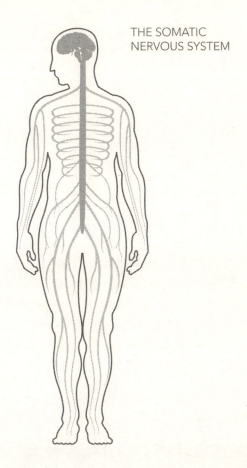

THE SOMATIC
NERVOUS SYSTEM

day. All of these things that we can't control but which control our lives.

All of these actions are controlled by something called the autonomic nervous system. This comprises two parts, the sympathetic nervous system and the parasympathetic nervous system. These have opposite actions to balance all of the various functions of the body; for example, the sympathetic nervous system makes the heart beat faster and the parasympathetic nervous system makes the heart beat slower.

EFFECTS OF THE AUTONOMIC
NERVOUS SYSTEM ON THE HEART

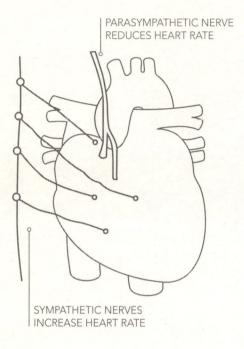

PARASYMPATHETIC NERVE
REDUCES HEART RATE

SYMPATHETIC NERVES
INCREASE HEART RATE

But it's much more complicated than that. This nervous system travels to every single organ in the body to control its actions. So when you become 'stressed', you can experience the typical reactions of:

- Dry mouth
- Shallow and rapid breathing
- Butterflies in the stomach, which signifies that the digestive process is slowing down
- Pale skin
- Sweating
- Fast heart rate

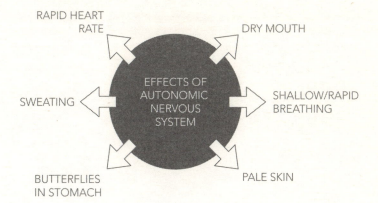

In other words, you are becoming agitated. This is fairly obvious when one becomes very agitated, but what is less obvious is the fact that this is happening in the body all the time to a varying degree, and having an effect on all of your organs and all of the systems in your body.

But how can this make you ill?

To answer this question, we need to look at all the major groups of illness to explain how they develop and how stress makes the process much, much worse. Because when you understand how this happens, you are then in a position to control it and prevent these ageing diseases from progressing to a certain degree.

Heart disease

In simple terms, heart disease is caused by insufficient blood carrying oxygen and food to the heart. This usually occurs because of blockage to the three arteries around the heart which can be due either to some sort of mechanical blockage (such as cholesterol) or to a restriction or narrowing of the coronary arteries occurring as a result of the nervous system causing stress.

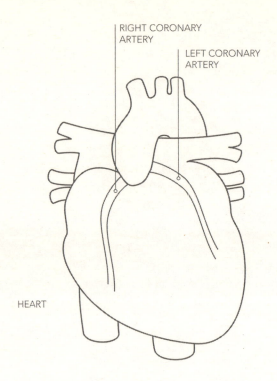

RIGHT CORONARY ARTERY

LEFT CORONARY ARTERY

HEART

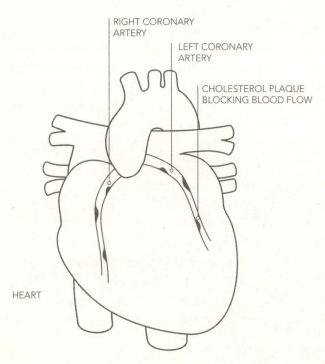

RIGHT CORONARY ARTERY

LEFT CORONARY ARTERY

CHOLESTEROL PLAQUE BLOCKING BLOOD FLOW

HEART

As will be explained later in this chapter, the nervous system can not only restrict the arteries around the heart, making them narrower and causing angina and possibly heart attacks, but it can also actually increase the level of cholesterol in the blood that blocks the arteries in the first place. So it is obvious that a significant controlling factor in heart disease is controlling the stress level of the body which can be done by relatively simple means. Not only will it prevent narrowing and blockage of the arteries, but it will also prevent the raised cholesterol that causes that blockage.

Diabetes

Diabetes is a condition which is affecting a greater proportion of the population every year. It is estimated that approximately 5% of the population have diabetes at present; however, as many as 24% may have a pre-diabetic condition called metabolic syndrome.

But why is diabetes important?

Because diabetes is the commonest cause of blindness in patients aged less than 65 years, and is a major cause of:

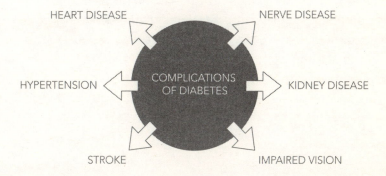

So obviously anything that causes diabetes, or contributes towards the cause of diabetes, is very important in the maintenance of health.

Stress makes diabetes worse, and can contribute to the development of diabetes. When you are stressed, organs in the back of the abdomen called the adrenal glands release a hormone called cortisol, which acts against another hormone called insulin, which can cause diabetes. So the more you are stressed, the more cortisol is produced, and therefore the more insulin is produced and therefore the worse diabetes becomes.

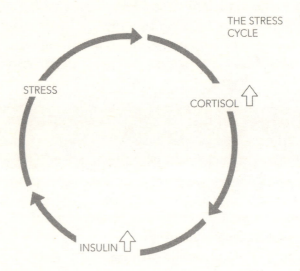

If diabetic control is poor, then blood sugar levels rise and, as explained in Chapter 2, blood sugar becomes incorporated into the body proteins and this causes wrinkling of the skin and weakening of structural proteins in the body such as blood vessels, which lead in turn to leaking of blood into the eye and into the nerves (see illustration on page 31).

It is absolutely essential to control blood sugar, and an important component of this process is to control stress levels.

Hypertension

Hypertension is the word we use for raised blood pressure. Obviously if the blood pressure rises too high then it can cause blood vessels to burst, such as in the brain which leads to a stroke, a weakness down one side of the body.

But why should blood pressure rise in the first place?

Obviously, if the heart beats faster and with greater force then this is likely to expand the blood vessels more and cause the blood pressure to increase, and, as we have seen, the cause of the heart beating faster and with greater force is stress stimulating the sympathetic nervous system by nerves which come from the brain and tell the heart to beat faster.

EFFECTS OF STRESS ON THE HEART

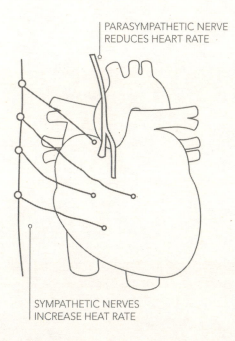

PARASYMPATHETIC NERVE
REDUCES HEART RATE

SYMPATHETIC NERVES
INCREASE HEAT RATE

So if you become agitated, the brain sends a message to the heart which stimulates it to beat faster and increases the blood pressure.

But there are other mechanisms for stress affecting blood pressure. All of the arteries in the body are controlled by nerves from the sympathetic nervous system which, when stimulated, constrict the vessels and make them narrower. Obviously, when a pump (the heart) has to push against a narrower vessel, the force that it needs is much higher and therefore the blood pressure rises.

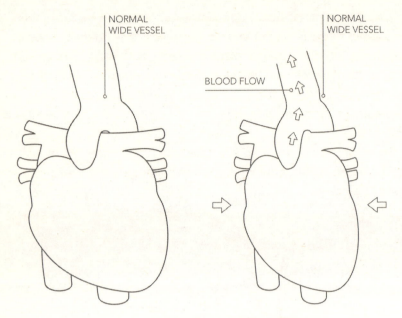

NORMAL
WIDE VESSEL

NORMAL
WIDE VESSEL

BLOOD FLOW

A. HEART PUMPS BLOOD AROUND BODY

EFFECTS OF HEART
PUMPING AGAINST NARROW ARTERIES

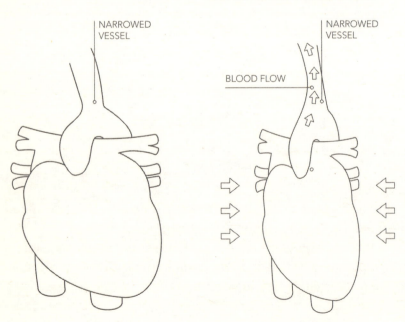

NARROWED
VESSEL

NARROWED
VESSEL

BLOOD FLOW

B. HEART NEEDS TO PUMP HARDER AGAINST NARROW VESSEL

So you can see that not only does the stress nervous system, the autonomic nervous system, cause the heart to beat faster but also the main arteries to be narrower, thereby increasing the pressure within those arteries. As will be described later in this chapter, stress can also increase the cholesterol levels in the blood, making the arteries even narrower and therefore increasing the blood pressure even further.

So, once again, you can see that reducing stress levels has a significant effect on reducing hypertension, and the side-effects of possible strokes.

High cholesterol

Everyone knows that you need to reduce your cholesterol level because otherwise it can cause heart disease and raised blood pressure. And the commonest way of reducing cholesterol is by using drugs called statins. But it is important to realise that statins affect only one part of this mechanism and that the underlying cause of raised cholesterol is increase in a hormone called insulin in the blood. And as we have seen, insulin is antagonised by the stress hormone cortisol, so if you become stressed the cortisol level rises and therefore the insulin level rises and therefore your cholesterol level rises.

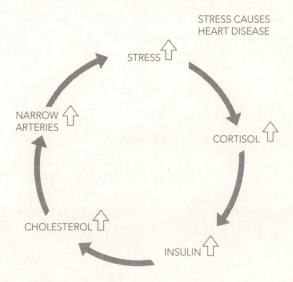

So, once again, it is absolutely essential to reduce the level of stress, in order to reduce blood cholesterol.

Stroke

The brain needs a constant supply of oxygen and nutrition from the arteries supplying it; a 'stroke' occurs when the blood flow to the brain is impaired in some way. This can be either by the artery being blocked, or the artery actually leaking due to increased blood pressure. We need to look at these two causes in detail to show how they develop, and how stress is a significant factor in their development.

1. Leaking blood vessel in the brain

If the pressure increases in any pipe, there is likely to be a leakage at any point where there is weakness in the pipe. This is simple plumbing. For example, if water freezes in a pipe, and expands, then it will burst the pipe when the water thaws. The simple answer to this is to lag or insulate the pipe and stop it happening.

Unfortunately, in the brain, the solution of lagging is not available. Essentially what happens is that the pressure of the blood vessels going into the brain becomes very high and, at a point of weakness, the blood vessel can break, causing a bleed into the nerve tissue and therefore a stroke. Obviously, the answer to this problem is simply to reduce the blood pressure and therefore reduce the likelihood of there being any leakage.

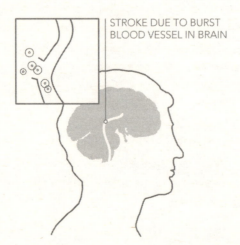

STROKE DUE TO BURST
BLOOD VESSEL IN BRAIN

2. Blocked blood vessel in the brain

The main cause of a blocked blood vessel is actually a blood clot travelling through an artery to the arteries of the brain and blocking one of the main arteries. But where does this blood clot come from? In most cases, the blood clot forms over an area of cholesterol in one of the blood vessels, either in the neck or in the valves of the heart. The blood vessel becomes slightly ruptured, and a clot forms in the surface to try to heal the vessel. But unfortunately a blood clot in an artery is very unstable as it can break off and flow into the artery to block somewhere, in this case commonly in the brain.

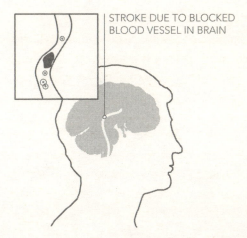

STROKE DUE TO BLOCKED
BLOOD VESSEL IN BRAIN

The ultimate origin of the blood clot is an area of narrowing of the blood vessel caused by cholesterol. And we know that raised cholesterol is significantly related to stress, so therefore reducing stress will reduce the likelihood of cholesterol plaques in the blood vessels, and therefore reduce the likelihood of blood clots forming on top of these plaques which can ultimately lead to a stroke.

It is therefore obvious that the two main causes of stroke, either the blood vessel bursting due to high blood pressure, or the blood vessel blocking due to blood clot, are both significantly related to increased stress levels and therefore will be significantly improved by reducing stress levels.

Peptic ulcer

Peptic ulcers are stomach ulcers which are caused, mainly, by stress. In essence, what happens is that the sympathetic nervous system (the stress nervous system) sends nerves, as we have said, to all the organs of the body, one of which is the stomach. The affect of stress on the stomach is to cause it to produce more acid, and although acid is essential to break down the food in your stomach, it can also cause some problems to the stomach lining if there is too much acid produced. So obviously, if the acid affects the lining of the stomach it can cause a breakdown and therefore an ulcer develops.

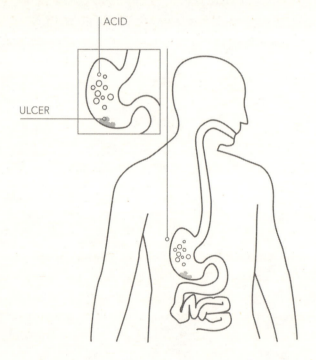

This causes indigestion, which is not very important, but it can also cause severe pain, and possibly, if the ulcer ruptures, it can cause death. It is essential to prevent the situation progressing to this stage and therefore reducing the acid in the stomach is very important.

There are many ways of reducing stomach acid, the easiest being by taking an antacid tablet, but this is like covering over the problem without actually addressing it. Ulcers can still develop if you take antacid tablets and the most important thing is to reduce the stress levels to prevent the ulcer from developing, or, if it has developed, to cause it to heal.

Back pain

Back pain is very common, and may be caused either by injury to the back or by protrusion of one of the discs in the back which presses on a nerve and causes severe pain, the classic 'slipped disc'.

Obviously, stress does not cause a slipped disc. The disc, between the bones of the back (called the vertebrae), can become weak with age and can rupture, causing pressure on a nerve and therefore pain.

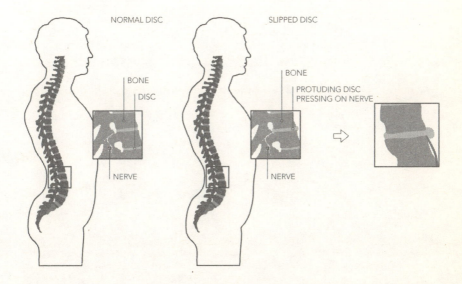

But the problem is that when pain develops, the muscles around the joint become very tense due to muscle spasm. This muscle spasm is directly caused by the stress of the pain causing the muscles to go into spasm.

When the muscle spasm occurs, it causes the bones to come closer together and therefore more pressure to be placed on the nerves. In other words, the initial slipped disc causes pressure on the nerve, this causes pain, and the pain (via the sympathetic nervous system) causes the muscles around the joint to go into spasm and press on the nerve even more.

MUSCLE IN SPASM
AROUND SLIPPED DISC

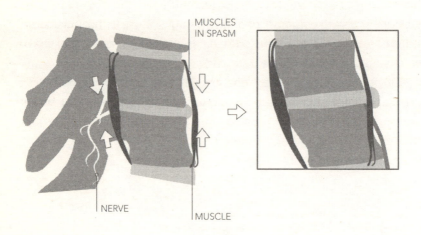

MUSCLES
IN SPASM

NERVE

MUSCLE

A vicious cycle develops of pain causing muscle spasm causing more pain.

THE VICIOUS CYCLE OF BACK PAIN

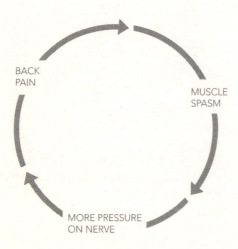

BACK
PAIN

MUSCLE
SPASM

MORE PRESSURE
ON NERVE

Therefore, by reducing the stress levels, one can reduce the muscle spasm and, although this does not cure the slipped disc, it relieves much of the pain caused by the secondary muscle spasm.

So reducing stress causes reduced muscle spasm and therefore reduces pain from a slipped disc.

Arthritis

There are many different forms of arthritis, but the commonest is osteoarthritis, which is caused primarily by ageing. In this particular form of arthritis, the cartilage over the joints becomes slightly worn away.

Bone surfaces must not come in contact with one another or it causes pain. To prevent this happening in the joints of the body there is a thin film of cartilage over the bones' surface and some 'oil' between the two surfaces to make them run smoothly.

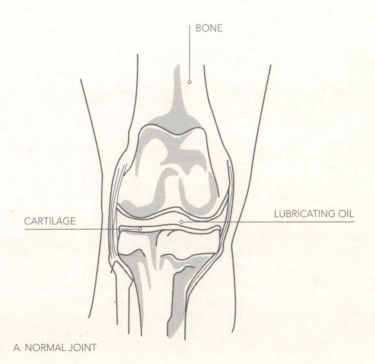

BONE

CARTILAGE

LUBRICATING OIL

A. NORMAL JOINT

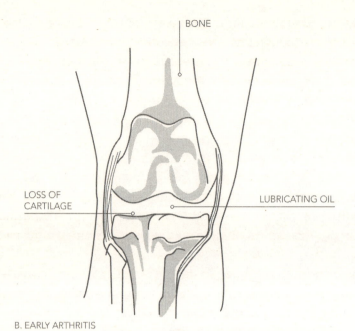

B. EARLY ARTHRITIS

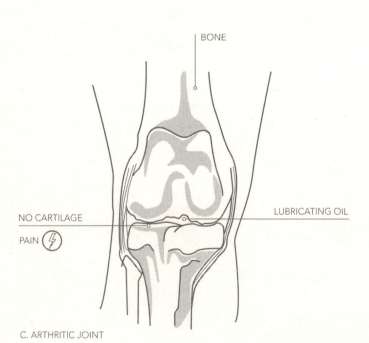

C. ARTHRITIC JOINT

As we age, the cartilage wears away and eventually the bone surfaces come in contact which causes pain. When bone surfaces rub against one another this causes quite severe pain, and once again, a vicious cycle develops where the pain stimulates muscle spasm around the joint, and the muscle spasm around the joint causes the bone surfaces to press even closer together causing more pain.

Obviously, as with back pain, the way to address this is to reduce the muscle spasm around the joint, allowing the bone surfaces to move slightly further apart and reduce the pain.

So you can see that although stress does not cause osteo-arthritis, it does cause the muscle spasm around the joint that makes the pain much worse. Reducing the stress levels reduces the muscle spasm and reduces the secondary pain.

The causes of stress

Stress, via the 'stress' hormones (adrenaline, cortisol) and the 'stress' nervous system (the autonomic nervous system), has many different diverse and potentially serious effects on physical health, from heart disease and strokes to diabetes and even exacerbating arthritis. In all of these ways, stress can cause significant reductions in the quality of life, even leading to potentially fatal illnesses.

We have seen how the stress hormones and the stress nervous system work, but what stimulates this reaction?

Stress comes from four main causes:

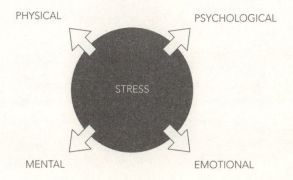

PHYSICAL   PSYCHOLOGICAL

STRESS

MENTAL   EMOTIONAL

- Physical, such as pain
- Psychological, from mental disturbances
- Emotional
- Mental

Whether stress is caused by physical, psychological or emotional reasons, the end result via the stress hormones and the stress nervous system is exactly the same, so essentially you can see that stress from any of these three causes has the same final effect, which is significant impairment of health.

As you can see, reduction in stress, and therefore reduction in the stress hormones and the reactions of the stress nervous system, are absolutely essential for health and are intrinsic to any form of preventive health system.

But how can you reduce these levels of stress in normal circumstances? In fact, this is relatively simple and, more importantly, completely inexpensive.

Stress is a fact of life. It

- cannot be avoided
- is usually associated with any change that requires adjustment
- is increased by negative feelings and poor coping reactions
- can be the result of major life changes or everyday hassles
- has both emotional and physical responses and consequences
- can be created internally by you or have external causes.

A certain level of stress helps everyone to function more efficiently. Too much stress, however, is counterproductive. It creates inefficiency, unpleasantness and is often mentally, physically and socially damaging. Stress that can be totally under your control is that caused by unrealistic expectations of yourself and/or others. Other stresses come from external realities that appear to be beyond control.

What matters crucially is your response!

To address and control the stress reaction you must initially obtain a measure of your own stress level.

Do you:

▓	eat balanced meals at regular intervals?	Y/N
▓	take regular exercise?	Y/N
▓	have a rhythm to your daily life?	Y/N
▓	have a pattern to your week?	Y/N
▓	drink no more than 1 unit of alcohol per day?	Y/N
▓	not smoke?	Y/N
▓	have and use a means of relaxation?	Y/N
▓	have a place at home where you can be undisturbed?	Y/N
▓	get enough sleep?	Y/N
▓	say 'No' to things you don't want to do?	Y/N
▓	deliberately avoid facing family problems?	Y/N

Score 1 point for every **Yes** answer and 0 points for every **No**.

Score: 0–5 points At high risk

6–10 points Some stress reduction required

11 points No problem

Lower than 6 points suggests that sudden extra pressure, whether good or bad, could send that stress up to the 'difficult to handle' level.

The secret to addressing stress problems is:

▓ recognising the signs as early as possible – only you know these

▓ taking time to assess the stress situations

▓ looking calmly at the pressures on you

▓ identifying any recent changes in your life

▓ noting recent changes in your feelings.

To manage stress effectively and systematically:

■ **Review your values and aims – start with the outcomes you want.**

■ **Act on the Alcoholics Anonymous mantra – identify the things that can be changed, accept those that cannot, have the wisdom to see the difference.**

■ **Throw away those attitudes, obligations and habits that stress you – and others.**

Many stresses are there because we are trapped by notions of what is right/ideal/always has been.

Having addressed the issues and redirected your *mental* approach to the problem, how can we combat the stress reaction by *physical* techniques?

1. Look after the important foundations of a balanced healthy life:

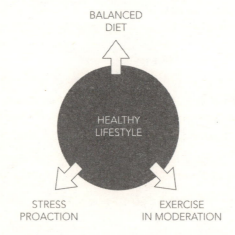

BALANCED
DIET

HEALTHY
LIFESTYLE

STRESS
PROACTION

EXERCISE
IN MODERATION

■ **Diet**

■ **Exercise**

■ **Reduce stress by directed mental approach**

2. Follow the three Rs:

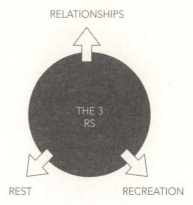

- **Relationships**
- **Recreation**
- **Rest**

3. Follow a physical programme to reduce stress hormones.

Controlling the autonomic nervous system

As you have already seen, the autonomic nervous system is the controlling mechanism for most of what you do and for maintaining your body on an even balance — which is the basis of good health. By its very definition, the autonomic nervous system is an 'automatic' system of regulation for all the functions of the body, such as heart rate, blood flow, breathing, digestion and so on. How can it be possible to control such an otherwise automatic nervous system, which is effectively in control of *you* for virtually all of your existence? There are essentially two different approaches to the control of stress, which are complementary rather than mutually exclusive: medical and non-medical.

Medical methods of controlling stress

While the autonomic nervous system (which determines our stress levels) is not the easiest mechanism to control by medical methods, it is certainly feasible with practice. And in an era of constant stress and pressures it is becoming more important to combat the adverse effects of stress on health.

One of the easiest ways to measure and assess autonomic control is by your heart rate, the rate at which your heart is beating. When you are relatively calm and relaxed, the heart beats at a smooth and even rate with few major fluctuations.

STABLE RESTING
HEART RATE

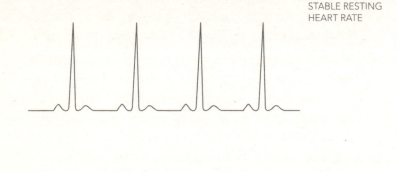

STRESSED
HEART RATE

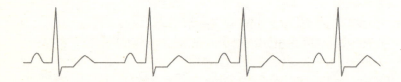

However, when you are stressed or anxious, your frustration is demonstrated most clearly by the heart rhythm, with marked variations in heart beats from fast to slow to irregular, producing a very disorganised general pattern.

The heart rate in this instance provides a very accurate measurement of how the autonomic controls of all the systems of your body are disturbed at the same time. We recognise this as stress and anxiety, but the body recognises it as a general imbalance of autonomic function which means that your bodily systems are not functioning smoothly.

So the secret to subjectively exerting a controlling influence on the autonomic nervous system is to control the heart rate. How can this be done? Well, as you might expect, the control of your body lies in your mind! Learning to control the autonomic nervous system is no more than an acquired and learned skill just like any other acquired skill. But it is not simple so don't expect instant results. Controlling your emotions and thoughts is a very difficult process but one which can definitely be achieved and which provides immense health benefits in the longer term.

There are five separate phases:

1. Preparation
   - **The basis of the programme is meditation, or just plain thinking about nothing. This is one of the most difficult exercises you can ever do as your mind is active at all times and you are always thinking of something, usually the problem which is causing the stress in the first place!**
   - **A second problem is that you need to eliminate all negative thoughts. This is much more difficult than you may realise as we are naturally negative in our thoughts, constantly worrying about situations that usually never happen!**
   - **Choose a peaceful time of day, when you can be undisturbed for at least 10 minutes, sit relaxed in a quiet room and close your eyes.**
   - **Concentrate on deep, even breathing, trying to achieve about 6–8 deep breaths per minute slowly.**
   - **Take 2–3 minutes of simple relaxing to achieve relative calm.**

2. Focus on the heart
   - **The next stage is to maintain focus on nothing! You need to release your mind from the traumas of everyday life – certainly not the easiest of objectives!**

▓ Try to concentrate on your heart beating in your chest. Just think about the heart and nothing else. This is a very difficult exercise, which is the reason why we have said 'try' because you are certainly not going to be successful initially. It really involves trying to empty your mind of everything else and focusing your concentration on one thing only, in this case the sensation of your heart beating slowly.

▓ Having concentrated on the heart for at least 2 minutes, you need to transfer your thoughts to your breathing, concentrating very specifically on breathing in and out at a steady, even pace.

▓ The rate at which you breathe has a significant effect on the heart rate. As you breathe in, the heart rate increases, and as you breathe out, the heart rate slows. This is very simply measured by taking your pulse at the same time as breathing slowly and deeply. Using the forefinger and middle finger of your right hand, take your pulse at the wrist of the left arm as shown:

TAKING THE PULSE
AT THE WRIST

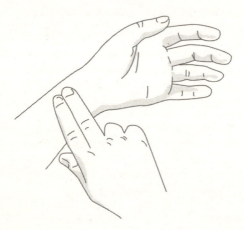

▓ Take a slow deep breath and you will notice your pulse increasing.

▓ Then continue the slow, even breathing rate and exhale slowly. You will notice the pulse rate slowing dramatically. This is the effect of the autonomic nervous system on the heart rate.

■ So if you can achieve reasonably even deep breaths, this will serve to stabilise your heart rate and make it more even, without the massive fluctuations which occur with anxiety and stress. In other words, what you are actually doing is controlling your stress level by concentrating specifically on breathing, which in turn controls heart rate.

3. Positive emotions

■ While maintaining a slow, deep and even rate of breathing, concentrate positively in an emotional sense about someone for whom you care. It is very important to try to eliminate all negative thoughts whenever they arise and to concentrate on one specific person. While this may seem a relatively simple technique, in practice you will find it very difficult indeed. The mind is constantly straying to negative thoughts, usually self-critical during periods of stress and anxiety, and you need to eliminate these destructive and negative emotions by concentrating on one specific idea. The most effective concept is usually someone for whom you most care. Although this is very difficult, you will eventually achieve this technique successfully, and will be much more relaxed in the process.

4. Achieving heart stability

■ Focus on one emotional thought for at least 2 minutes, concentrate on breathing at a slow even rate of 6 breaths per minute (which is quite slow) and focusing specifically on the one thought. All the time, particularly when you are beginning the heart-focus method, your brain will be hyperactive and constantly straying to other subjects but each time this happens try to concentrate on one person and bring your attention back to focus.

5. Reconnect slowly

■ After approximately 2 minutes, and this seems a very long time when you are sitting still and thinking of one thought only, concentrate once again, on a steady breathing rate for about **30 seconds**, slowly and evenly, then concentrate once again on the heart rate.

▨ Transfer your concentration to the beating of your heart, thinking of your heart and nothing else for at least **1–2 minutes**, and then slowly open your eyes and relax.

This is an extremely difficult exercise to perform, and it will take some months before you can achieve it perfectly. It would seem remarkably simple to sit and think about nothing, or to concentrate on your heart or your breathing, but In actual fact your mind is constantly thinking negative thoughts during periods of stress and anxiety and it takes some time to achieve this. However, when you are successful, you are beginning to control your autonomic nervous system and you will notice much more peaceful periods in your life even though there may be considerable external stresses.

If you control the negative effects of the autonomic system during stress, it is obvious that this can have significant effects on cardiac function and therefore on preventing heart disease by preventing stressful constriction of the coronary arteries.

EFFECTS OF STRESS
ON THE HEART

RIGHT CORONARY
ARTERY

LEFT CORONARY
ARTERY

CHOLESTEROL PLAQUE
BLOCKING BLOOD FLOW

INCREASED
HEART RATE

INCREASED
BLOOD PRESSURE

HEART

CONSTRICTION OF
CORONARY ARTERY

However, what is not so obvious is the effect it will have on so many other functions controlled by stress, such as arthritis with tension of the muscles due to muscle spasm around joints.

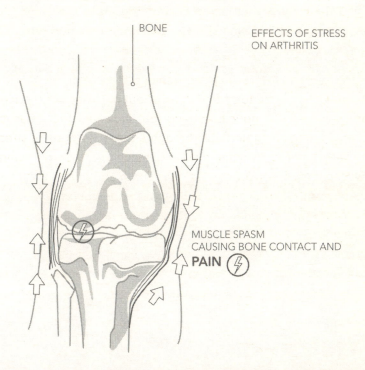

BONE

EFFECTS OF STRESS
ON ARTHRITIS

MUSCLE SPASM
CAUSING BONE CONTACT AND
PAIN

Or much less obvious mechanisms like the immune system, which controls our reactions to infection and cancer. As we have already mentioned, the stress mechanism in the body has widespread adverse effects, although it can also have good effects on our body in terms of preparing us to deal with difficult situations.

Although you can perform autonomic exercises with no special-ised equipment, this technique can actually be measured by an objective and visual method. Often it can be easier to control emotions when you can actually *see* the effects of your actions and receive an immediate positive feedback.

The programme which measures heart rate in relation to auto-nomic stress is called HeartMath. It demonstrates on a computer the heart rate rhythms while you are performing these techniques. It also shows you in terms of very simple visual stimuli (such as red, amber and green lights) how you are moving from areas of high stress, which are obviously red, to those of high relaxation and heart rate control, which are coloured green. Many people find that pictorial representation — by actually seeing the changes in heart rate in this way — can help them to achieve this, and it is undoubtedly a very successful technique. However, there is some expense involved and it is certainly not essential for controlling the autonomic nervous system which can be performed simply and effectively at no cost whatsoever.

If you are interested in following this further I suggest you look up www.heartmath.com which explains the practicalities of the technique. It is simply achieved by using an external heart rate monitor which attaches to the body and is then controlled via a computer. It can also be achieved via a small handheld monitor.

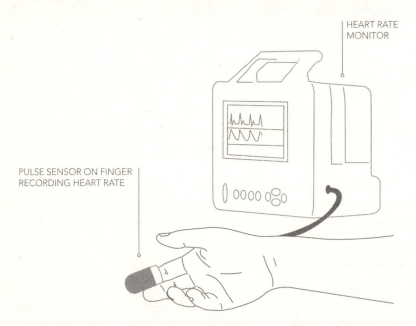

HEART RATE
MONITOR

PULSE SENSOR ON FINGER
RECORDING HEART RATE

In summary you can now appreciate that, although the autonomic nervous system controls the whole of the body and is the only responsible mechanism for stress within the body, it can be controlled (to some degree) externally by specific techniques to exercise the mind rather than the body. Many of our current techniques are actually based upon ancient tradition! In particular, meditation techniques have been with us for thousands of years, all achieving the same effect of controlling the autonomic nervous system and reducing stress.

One cannot emphasise enough the importance of stress reduction in not only achieving peace of mind, but also in the prevention and control of many physical illnesses.

Physical approaches to disease without addressing the mental aspect will never be entirely successful.

Non-medical methods of controlling stress

Of course, although medical techniques for relieving stress are well documented and have unequivocal medical effects, there are many non-medical approaches to stress relief which, although with less stringent medical credentials, nevertheless have proven effectiveness in this regard. It is well to remember that alternative techniques are merely 'those which are not within the realms of conventional medicine'. Massage (in its many varieties), aromatherapy, acupuncture, yoga and meditation are just a few of the myriad of techniques which have been effectively employed in stress relief. In fact, acupuncture was widely ridiculed before the medical discovery of endorphins, the body's natural opiates, which are stimulated by acupuncture techniques.

In the Programme (page 92), several natural techniques are described in the 'winding down' phase of the day. Stress relief takes many forms, the only important aspect being to relieve stress by whatever non-invasive and safe method is suitable to the individual!

5 The importance of water

THE HUMAN BODY is made primarily of water! This would seem obvious. However, matters which are obvious occasionally become lost in the mists of time and we forget to place as much emphasis on them as we should as we grow older. Babies are made up of 85% water, but as we age the amount of water in our bodies tends to lower, primarily as a result of dehydration caused by ourselves! In other words, we simply don't drink enough water for *optimal* health: we actually tend to only consume sufficient fluid to function. The average adult has a water content of over 75%; however, in those over 70 years old this can reduce to 65% for men and 52% for women.

Death occurs at water levels of only 10% lower than this!

So you can appreciate the absolute necessity of drinking water on a regular basis for health. The normal situation is to drink water when we need it, when we are thirsty. However, by that stage our body water levels are becoming dangerously low; the body is dehydrated and the brain is crying out for water. In actual fact, for health we need to drink water *before we need it*! In other words, the secret is to prevent dehydration and its problems, rather than wait for dehydration to occur.

In fact, the benefits of drinking water *before* becoming thirsty are probably higher than any other health benefit of diet, exercise or stress. We just don't think to drink water throughout the day. We wait for our body to tell us that we are thirsty by which time the brain has become clinically dehydrated. Your body is in fact remarkably resilient. When we become slightly dehydrated, or dry, it will actually conserve water from some of the less important parts of the body. This is quite obvious when you think of not passing as much urine or developing constipation due to dehydration; it is less obvious when water is conserved from all the other cells in the body. The body has 50 trillion cells (50,000,000,000,000), each of which contains approximately 75% water. All of the bodily functions depend on water for lubrication.

Dehydration affects every system in the body and can have profound effects on the most common diseases. Let us examine the systems that can be affected by dehydration. We will look at the obvious systems initially, such as urinary tract and kidney function, then examine the less obvious afterwards. I have no doubt that you will identify medical problems which relate specifically to your current situation.

Kidney function

One of the more obvious effects of dehydration is the colour of your urine. Not quite so obvious is the fact that if urine has *any* colour then it is concentrated. In other words, normal urine should be colourless and odourless. If the urine is coloured, the body is concentrating its urine to preserve water which is totally unnecessary. The kidney's job is to remove the toxins from the body. The darker the colour of urine, the more toxins, and the more you need to drink to return it to the healthy colourless state.

Bowel function

Everyone is aware of the importance of fibre in our diet to improve digestion. Fibre is found in many foods such as vegetables, multi-grain bread and fruit. It travels down the digestive tract, stretching it and stimulating the bowel to keep the food travelling and prevent it becoming static – or dehydrated. It is precisely this stretching which keeps the bowel moving.

What is less commonly understood is that the lubrication for this process is water! Approximately two pints (1 litre) of water are lost during every healthy bowel motion. So in other words, the easiest way to keep the bowels moving is to drink more water. As unhealthy bowel motions are associated significantly with bowel cancer and bowel inflammatory diseases, this is the way to reduce the likelihood of these complications developing.

Mental fatigue and tiredness

The brain consists of 85% water in a baby and 75% water in an adult. As we have seen, this may drop to less than 60% in those who are older, and the brain depends entirely upon water to function. The nervous system controls all our voluntary and involuntary actions, so if the brain becomes dehydrated, many essential bodily functions are affected. The most obvious effect is fatigue but this is merely one of many symptoms. So drink regularly to keep the brain functioning at optimal levels!

Indigestion

Indigestion is primarily caused by acid reflux in the stomach. The stomach contains concentrated acid and if you consider the matter (and it is not that difficult), the more water you have in the stomach, the less concentrated the acid and the less likely it will be to cause indigestion. In other words, acid reflux, the cause of peptic ulcers, *will be reduced by simply drinking more water and diluting the acid in your stomach.*

Muscle pains

The commonest cause of muscle pain is a build-up of a substance called lactic acid in the muscles due to exertion. As with all other problems, when this is 'washed out' by drinking more water, the lactic acid levels are diluted and the muscle pains are inevitably less.

Arthritis (particularly rheumatoid arthritis)

As we have explained earlier, arthritis is primarily caused by joint surfaces being in apposition with one another, in other words, touching one another (see Illustration, page 52). Joint surfaces should never touch otherwise pain will occur. To prevent the joint surfaces from actually touching one another, a thin layer of oil is situated between the joint surfaces which lubricates the surfaces and keeps them moving smoothly. Arthritis has a major correlation with dehydration as the cartilage in the joints contains water and when the water in the body level decreases, the cartilage levels may touch. In other words, when you are dehydrated the body gives priority to various structures (such as the brain) to maintain the fluid levels of those structures. To do so, it must favour some tissues at the expense of others – and some of the least prioritised are the joints. The cartilage between joints can therefore become more abrasive and inflammation can occur, with inevitable pain which we call arthritis.

However, some of the more important causes of medical problems resulting from dehydration are much less obvious. We have already seen that the major causes of ageing are:

- raised levels of blood sugar
- raised stress levels
- high cholesterol

But these are in fact intrinsically related to increasing dehydration. There are many reasons why dehydration causes significant medical problems:

- **Stress**

  Stress is integrally associated with the level of hydration of the body. In other words, when the level of fluid in the body decreases, the level of stress will inevitably increase. Remember the brain is 85% pure water in a baby, and 75% in an adult. Dehydration of only one or two percentage points has a major effect on the way the brain deals with information from multiple inputs. Any reduction in the brain's capacity to handle stress can lead to depression and mood swings. For example, low blood sugar causes significant depression of mood, leading to stress.

Much more importantly, there are significant objective medical effects when the body becomes dehydrated. Cortisol (the stress hormone) is released primarily into the body when it is stressed or dehydrated.

Raised blood cholesterol

There are many reasons why cholesterol levels elevate during periods of stress. As we have seen, dehydration of the body causes cortisol levels to increase and this inevitably works against insulin and raises blood cholesterol and blood triglycerides, a significant factor in the development of heart disease. However, in a more simplistic way, the level of cholesterol in the blood inevitably increases simply because the proportion of cholesterol is higher during dehydration than it would be in a fully hydrated state. In other words, if you have 100% water in the body, and there is 5% cholesterol, then the cholesterol is 5%; if there is 50% water and cholesterol level is 5% then the cholesterol level is artificially elevated to 10% because of the dehydration. So the same amount of cholesterol makes up a higher proportion in a dehydrated patient, who therefore has a much higher risk of developing arterial disease and heart disease than someone fully hydrated. One of the secrets to lower blood cholesterol levels is to drink enough water.

How do we prevent dehydration?

First of all, the most important thing is *don't cause the problem*! There are several factors in life that can exacerbate dehydration significantly. The most obvious is not drinking sufficient water; we will return to that in a moment. The less obvious are the lifestyle factors that can cause significant dehydration and significant disease. These factors are:

- **excess alcohol intake**
- **excess caffeine intake**
- **carbonated drinks**
- **smoking**
- **dietary imbalance between cooked foods and raw foods**

Alcohol leads to dehydration by suppressing a hormone in the body called vasopressin. In other words, if you drink much alcohol, you will become dehydrated unless you also drink a large amount of water.

Caffeine (and other alkaloid stimulants) cause dehydration. You don't need to exclude coffee, merely drink less!

Strangely, excessive exercise can cause increased insulin production and dehydration. In other words, if you exercise, then make sure that you drink copious amounts of fluid to compensate.

- **Hot dry climates cause dehydration, so drink more fluids. Not exactly rocket science!**
- **Airline travel causes extreme dehydration; drink more on long flights.**
- **Sugar: in association with its role as a major problem of ageing, sugar also causes significant dehydration (which causes more ageing) because every molecule of sugar uses one molecule of water to break it down to two molecules of glucose.**
- **Smoking causes dehydration. If you must smoke, drink more, or better still don't smoke!**

How much water to drink

There may be statements made such as 'you should drink eight glasses of water a day'; however, this is completely wrong. Why?

Because we are all different, we have different lifestyles and different requirements. Basically the amount of water that you require depends on what your activity is and what your lifestyle entails. If you include any of the previous activities in your daily lifestyle, then you will need to consume even more water.

However, the absolute minimum amount of water you require is the equivalent (in ounces) of half your body weight (in pounds). This sounds very complicated but it is actually very simple; 8 oz (226 g) equals one cup, so a 160 lb (72 kg) person would require a minimum of 10 cups of water (80 oz/2.2 kg) per day. In effect, a typical male or female will require at least 10 cups of water per day, in addition to any other fluids he or she may drink.

This fluid intake per day does not include tea, coffee or soft drinks (and particularly not alcohol) but rather just pure water in addition to anything else you may drink. Do so and you will increase your hydration levels dramatically – and reduce the risk of premature ageing!

6 Spring into action

EXERCISE!

If exercise is not for you then read no further. However, if you wish to obtain the maximum benefit from this programme and develop a supple and toned body then read on.

Have you ever taken time to consider just how much wear and tear your body has suffered over the years? Everyday life takes a tremendous toll on the body in ways that you would probably not realise. Busy lifestyles lead to excessive stresses on joints. And many of the problems are caused by poor posture:

- Starting at the basic support for your body, your feet, with ill-fitting shoes, which affect not only your feet, but entire muscle balance throughout the body
- Incorrect posture carrying children
- Poor posture in the workplace, particularly at the office desk
- Poor posture while driving, causing neck tension
- Posture implications for the spine when lifting heavy items, such as furniture, and while gardening, etc.

The list is endless. In fact, for most of us, for most of our lifetimes, poor posture is the norm, not the exception. And as posture determines our muscle balance in almost every situation, it is absolutely essential to get the balance right to prevent arthritis developing later in life.

If you recognise the above signs, making simple adjustments to your attitude and lifestyle to exercise would certainly increase your standard of life, and possibly also your length of life.

This programme is very different from any other you have encountered. It won't involve complicated aerobic exercises, special equipment, exorbitant cost on gym fees or personal trainers — or even much time!

However, before we proceed, you really have to understand the purpose of exercise. That would seem fairly obvious: the purpose of exercise is to be slimmer and look better.

No, it's not!

The purpose of exercise is to make you healthier. It will not make you slimmer because when you exercise you inevitably eat more. So initially, we have to understand the purpose of what you are actually doing.

To do this is to go back to the basics of the body structure. The body is essentially an underlying framework, like scaffolding, made of bone: the skeleton. This is the basis of our support.

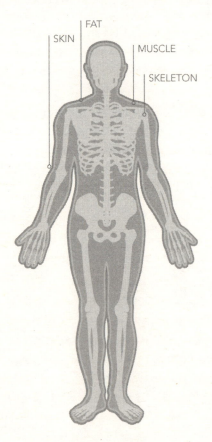

Overlying the skeleton is a layer of muscle, then a layer of fat and finally the outer covering of skin. So it is fairly easy to appreciate that by reducing the fat layer you will become slimmer. However, it is also easily appreciated that if you tone the muscle layer you will assume a much better toned body shape. So you will lose the overlying layer of fat, the cellulite, and have a toned body structure because of the muscle tone beneath.

But, of course, as with everything, it is not as simple as that. The muscles have to be exercised in some way to increase their tone and also to increase their flexibility. There is absolutely no point in increasing the power and strength in the muscles without their being flexible and able to stretch. So, in simple terms, we have to initially map our own body to work out the problem areas and to deal with those appropriately. First of all, we need to identify the landmarks of the body and how to increase their tone and flexibility:

- **Feet**
- **Knees**
- **Hip bones and pelvis**
- **Ribs**
- **Shoulders**
- **Head and neck**

Essentially this is a programme based upon three main principles:

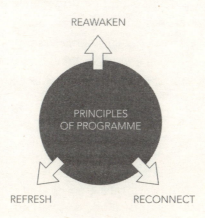

REAWAKEN

PRINCIPLES
OF PROGRAMME

REFRESH   RECONNECT

- Reawaken
- Reconnect
- Refresh

Reawaken

The first thing we should do is to reawaken dormant muscles by stretching and strengthening and improving their flexibility.

Reconnect

You have to reconnect with your body as the first stage of moving forward. When was the last time you actually considered your body? Probably never! Stretching your muscles in small stages is a good start. When you bend initially, maybe your fingers will only touch your knees the first day but every day you will reach a few millimetres lower with ease. The importance is to try.

Unfortunately, bad habits are a natural association with age. We become lazy; a typical example is poor posture when driving. Not necessary but it is what we do. In the same way, we can develop less mobility by adopting poor movements in our joints and muscles in every action of the body. This basically develops because of lack of use and being unaware of your own body's needs and requirements. It is possible for us to blame our inability to reconnect with our bodies on our lifestyle and work commitments, however the bottom line is that we need to make a reconnection. Over a period of many years, we become less flexible and our muscles and joints deteriorate. However, the important thing to realise is that you can actually halt and in many cases reverse this process substantially by taking control.

Refresh

Once have *reconnected* with your body, you can begin to refresh your lifestyle. Initially, you need to evaluate yourself and your lifestyle and what actually motivates you. An effective stretching routine, followed by exercises, must be part of your lifestyle.

Having evaluated the situation, the next stage is motivation. An effective stretching routine must be part of your lifestyle for improved quality of life, which is the whole basis of health. But it has to be realistic.

Set your own goals

The initial stage is to set realistic targets within a realistic time frame. There is no point expecting to be an Olympic athlete within a week because it just is not going to happen. But you can improve your shape and flexibility within a realistic time frame and improve your standard of life. So initially, you need to evaluate the body shape you want and can reasonably expect to achieve in a given period of time.

Incentive

Incentive is entirely up to you. If it is not there you're not going to feel motivated. It does not cost anything and it is easy to achieve so let's go for it.

Set aside time

Time is the only thing that you have in life – and the only concept you have to lose! It comes and goes but it is yours to decide what you want to do with it, particularly when you are over 50. Set aside a small amount of time for your daily stretching and exercise routine and it will happen. The common statement that people make is 'I just don't have time'. Of course you have time. Take away 10 minutes from reading the newspaper and there is the time.

The right time

However, as important as setting aside time is setting aside the *correct* time for your daily exercise, particularly when you are over 50.

There is no point in planning an exercise regime at 6.30am if you do not regularly rise at 6.30am. Set aside a time that is suitable for you and stick to it.

Plan your sessions

Choose a different exercise every few sessions. Again, there is no point in repeating the same exercise over and over again until you have mastered it. The aim is to improve the fitness of your whole body, not just a section. Many people make the mistake of only exercising one or two muscle groups, for example biceps, and it just does not work. This exercise regime will give you a full and complete plan in a few minutes a day, with excellent results. Choose a different exercise every few sessions.

Explore the range of movement you are capable of and look for vulnerable areas. The secret is to improve the weak areas, not the ones that you are good at. If you feel tension in one or more muscle groups, you may wish to concentrate on that, starting slowly at first and gradually building up. Initially you may feel rather awkward, but that is natural. Anyone who has not done exercise for several years, or often many years, will be awkward. But the main thing is that you are going to achieve your desired aim and that is all that is important. You do not need to worry about looking silly because you are looking silly in your own home with nobody seeing you. At the end of the day, you are going to be flexible and fit and certainly not look silly. In other words, you have reconnected with your body and you will be refreshed.

Simplicity

Simplicity is the main element when setting out your stretching routine. This involves time: choose the right time for you, either morning, afternoon or evening.

Place: A quiet spot in your house or even in the garden
Clothing: Relaxed, comfortable and loose
Music: Soft and soothing, always helps

Observe what happens to your body when you complete a stretching routine. Take note of the small improvements and be revitalised and refreshed, and much more important feel confident.

Timing

Remember that fitness cannot be worked on just two days a week alone. An effective exercise programme must be part of your daily routine and you must enjoy it. First evaluate yourself and your lifestyle and motivate yourself, set goals and rewards, establish priorities, work out a schedule and choose those physical activities you enjoy most.

As previously stated, wear comfortable clothing. Don't push yourself too far. Stretching is the most important component of exercise because as we age our muscles become shorter and tauter and without stretching they are more susceptible to knee, hip, shoulder and elbow injuries, many of which you may already have. This is going to make them better by reducing muscle spasm around the painful joints and increasing flexibility. Stretching can be incorporated into everything you do.

Breathing

I know that it seems rather obvious as we all breathe, but breathing is probably one of the most important things we do. Relaxation occurs at a maximum of six breaths per minute, which is actually very, very slow. What we need to do is to learn to relax so that our breathing controls the relaxation of our muscles.

Don't expect instant results

Instant results just are not going to happen. Remember, you are reversing something that has happened over the last 30 years so it is going to take some time to get there. But you will get there and you will feel better and you will feel refreshed and reconnect with your body.

In short, you are incorporating a complete plan with nutrition, mental health and practical self-awareness, which culminates in physical fitness, commensurate with your age.

Once again, let's begin

All exercise – of whatever nature – has basically three objectives: to improve

- **Muscle tone**
- **Power**
- **Coordination**

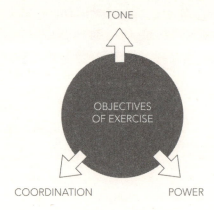

It is essential to address all three; concentrating on any one aspect at the expense of the others results in imbalance and stress to the body. For example, if you perform exclusively power exercises, this will impair coordination. The details of the exercise regime are described in the Programme (pages 96–137); however, the principles are as follows.

The basis of all exercise regimes should be BALANCE, by which we mean muscle balance. All muscles have a specific function, and for every muscle there is another muscle which does the opposite, thus preserving muscle balance. It is absolutely essential to exercise muscles in groups to ensure the maintenance of this balance or the result will be ineffective. This programme has been specifically developed to maintain that balance for maximal effect.

Stretching exercises for shoulders and chest (page 96)

This is an excellent stretching exercise for the upper body, and, most importantly, involves very little straining. It is absolutely essential in any form of exercise to avoid straining and excessive exertion at the beginning, and you will be amazed how quickly the results will be achieved thereafter.

The most important aspect of any exercise regime is posture.

Posture is the basis of your body's entire muscle coordination. Your body requires equal balance on each side of the body; if posture is poor, this will result in muscle imbalance, which in turn causes muscle spasm, exacerbating any arthritic changes which are present. So you can realise that it is absolutely essential to maintain muscle balance by good posture in all situations. These exercises are designed specifically to prevent muscle imbalance and prevent muscle spasm – which is one of the commonest causes of pain.

Chest and bust exercise (page 100)

Muscles of the chest and upper back are often not exercised in normal usage and therefore can become weak. As these are the muscles that hold up the shoulder girdle, it is obviously essential that we exercise these in moderation. This does not require expensive gym equipment but can be done very simply sitting at your desk or in an easy chair.

Upper back exercise (page 114)

Whenever you exercise one group of muscles it is absolutely essential to exercise those that work against them, and in this case it is the upper back muscles. So having exercised the chest we need to exercise the upper back muscles which pull the shoulder girdle back. Once again this is very simply done with no equipment.

The upper arms (page 106)

Upper arm exercises are very important because they control much of the power of the arms and are very simple to perform safely and effectively.

Balance (pages 102 and 103)

One of the most important exercises which is frequently forgotten is that of balance. When we balance we are using virtually all of the muscles of the trunk and the legs which are controlling our every movement and preventing us from falling over. This would seem a relatively simple exercise, but in fact when you take one leg away the whole difficulty of the balance situation becomes much more apparent. However, it does exercise so many muscle groups in a gentle way that it is absolutely essential.

Upper thighs and bottom (page 110)

The reason why this area has commonly poor muscle tone is because it is seldom exercised! You may think that you exercise this area when you sit down but in actual fact nothing happens unless you actively stretch the muscles. This is a relatively simple exercise which has an immense effect on improving muscle tone in this very obvious area.

Once again, as with all muscle exercises, it is important to exercise the muscles which work against those on each side of the body. So having exercised the muscles on the back of the leg, it is essential to exercise those on the front of the leg to balance muscle tone throughout the body. This exercises both the top part of the leg in the front, and also the calves.

Hips and thighs (page 98)

Fat is stored on the hips primarily because of the hormone insulin, and if you follow the dietary programme on pages 97–137 then this fat deposition will be reversed and you will remove this unsightly bulge. However, it is also important to increase the muscle tone underneath the fat layer as obviously the muscles around the hip joint play a very important part in controlling muscle tone and preventing arthritis.

This exercise uses a fitness ball and an exercise mat, which are very easily obtained and relatively inexpensive. This is a very safe exercise which allows you to tone the muscles around the hips without placing any strain on the hips whatsoever. To perform this exercise, you will be lying flat on the floor and therefore relieving all the pressure from the joint and therefore can be performed safely by patients with arthritis.

The advantage of this exercise is that it tones the muscles around the hip, a very difficult joint to exercise in isolation, while placing no pressure on it whatsoever. Any exercise which involves standing erect obviously places considerable strain on the hip, and if there are any arthritic changes this can be quite dangerous. In this exercise all of the pressure is removed and the muscles are therefore relaxed while performing the exercise.

Abdomen and tummy (page 126)

It is important to perform this exercise causing as little strain as possible to the abdominal muscles, which are usually very poorly developed! The abdomen and tummy muscles are very important to exercise, not just from the cosmetic perspective but also the fact that they are the muscles which act in the opposite direction of your upper back muscles – but once again, you must always exercise muscles on both sides of the body at the same time.

Waistline (page 122)

This simple exercise for the waistline is an excellent adjunct to the previous exercise. It involves virtually no stress whatsoever, and is perfectly safe. For this exercise, you need the fitness ball once again.

Neck exercises (page 128)

One of the most important (and commonly overlooked) areas is the neck. The neck supports the head, a rather obvious statement, but it is important to remember that neck strain can cause significant arthritis of the neck, a risk that can be significantly reduced by muscle tone in this area. Once again, it is essential to exercise each of the muscle groups separately to obtain muscle balance for all of the muscle groups around the neck.

Initially we have to exercise the muscles moving the head forwards and backwards, then from side to side.

Tension release (pages 130 and 131)

This is a very gentle muscle release tension exercise; however, it has the added advantage of increasing generalised muscle tone, which is otherwise difficult to achieve by separating the muscle groups. This is often most usefully performed at the end of any exercise regime. Tension is commonly relieved by stimulating the sole of the foot, as demonstrated by such techniques as massage and aromatherapy.

Walking

And last, but by no means least, is walking, the most effective exercise of all. Twenty minutes' walking – at normal walking pace – on three occasions per week has been shown to have immense health benefits in terms of circulation. Enjoy walking outdoors – not on a treadmill – and you have all the added advantages of fresh air! So walk regularly for improved health and vitality!

7 Case studies

OF COURSE IT is very simple to make sweeping statements about the advantages of following a particular programme, but can they be proved?

Fortunately, in our clinic we have treated thousands of people with this system and all have been assessed by objective medical measures. In other words, standard principles applied to the various conditions in medicine have been applied in these cases: measurements of blood sugar and insulin in diabetes, obviously measurement of cholesterol profiles in patients with heart disease and raised cholesterol, and an assessment of insulin in patients who are predisposed to diabetes but have not yet developed the condition.

It is probably most appropriate to look at the various conditions individually, such as diabetes, raised cholesterol and heart disease, and then to examine the ways in which this programme has significantly improved the medical condition. However, it is equally important to realise that these conditions do not occur in isolation: in other words, patients with type 2 diabetes (the type of diabetes associated with ageing) will also have raised cholesterol and insulin levels – not just increases in blood sugar – and will also be overweight. Patients with raised cholesterol levels are also likely to have raised insulin levels and be liable to diabetes, simply because insulin is one of the commonest factors in the development of cholesterol problems.

Patients with heart disease will, in most cases, have raised cholesterol and raised insulin levels, predisposing to diabetes. Many are overweight because of their raised insulin levels.

This is not intended to confuse you, but rather to explain that most of these conditions are actually completely interrelated. They do not stand in isolation and they are not separate conditions. Medicine does not work that way; most conditions in medicine are interrelated with other conditions and don't stand in isolation. But the important part is that when you control one you will control all! And that is the central point of this book. The importance of trying to control 'ageing' is that *you have to deal with a number of situations at the same time*. However, as they are mainly interrelated it is relatively simple to do so.

Let us examine some common conditions to see the effect of the programme.

Diabetes

CASE STUDY 1

George is a 47-year-old driving instructor and had been newly diagnosed with type 2 diabetes. He had noticed extreme tiredness for several months, a change in his eyesight, a dry mouth and lethargy. This was particularly important, as his job as a driving instructor meant that he had to be alert at all times. He had tried the usual treatments, and was on diabetic and cholesterol medication, as his blood results were as follows:

- Blood sugar 12.2 (normal is less than 5.8 mmol/l)
- Cholesterol level 7.6 (normal is less than 4–5 mmol/l)
- Glycosylated haemoglobin (HbA1c) 12.5 (normal is less than 6.5%)

Glycosylated haemoglobin is the measure of long-term control of diabetes.

So it can be seen that although George was newly diagnosed with diabetes, his readings were in fact quite catastrophic. With a blood sugar level over twice the normal and a very high cholesterol level, his risk of developing severe diabetic complications and heart disease was very high.

Within one month of commencing the Age Revolution Programme, addressing his nutrition, exercise and stress levels, George's weight had reduced by 5 kg (11 lb) from 84 kg (185 lb) to 79 kg (174 lb). His blood sugar level had reduced to 6.0 (i.e. almost normal). His glycosylated haemoglobin had reduced from 12.4 to 6.1 (i.e. normal) and his cholesterol measure had reduced from 7.5 to 3.0 (normal). In other words, he had completely controlled the diabetes and cholesterol level by lifestyle management. At this point obviously there were concerns regarding his medication and we began to reduce the medication appropriately.

This is not just an isolated case, but rather a common event which is seen on many occasions. Application of the principles of the Age Revolution Programme reduces the effects of newly diagnosed type 2 diabetes, which may then be controlled without medication in many cases.

This is hardly surprising when you consider that the prevalence of diabetes has increased by 4–5 times over the past 20 years, which obviously cannot be due to genetic causes, as our genes have not changed in 20 years, and therefore it is due to lifestyle. While this in itself is a very concerning phenomenon, obviously if something can be caused by lifestyle then it can be equally reversed by lifestyle, and that is exactly what is happening in this case.

CASE STUDY 2

Mary was a 61-year-old patient with poorly controlled type 2 diabetes. She was having severe difficulty with losing weight – in fact couldn't avoid increasing weight for much of her life. She had recently retired as a teacher, but had such low energy levels that she was unable to enjoy her retirement. When she presented to the clinic, she was on maximal oral diabetic medication and anti-cholesterol medication, which was still failing to control her diabetes and cholesterol levels, and it was likely that she would need to be commenced on insulin, which she did not want! Her fasting blood glucose was 8.3 mmol/l (normal 5.8) and her fasting cholesterol level was 6.2 mmol/l (normal less than 5). She weighed 90 kg (198 lb) and her weight was increasing. Her insulin level was 12.7 (normal 5.0 mIU/l). As insulin is the hormone which controls your weight, it was impossible for Mary to reduce weight with such a high insulin level. Insulin is controlled by the amount of carbohydrates in your diet and stress levels (pages 41–42).

Within one week of commencing the programme, Mary's blood sugar levels began to drop dramatically, and it was necessary to reduce her medication for diabetes by 50%. This was reduced by a further 25% within a week. Within one month of the programme, on only 25% of the medication she was taking previously, Mary's blood sugar had reduced from 8.3 mmol/l to 5.5 mmol/l (normal). Her cholesterol level reduced to 4.5 mmol/l (normal) and her insulin level had reduced from 12.7 mmol/l to 7.5 (almost normal). Weight had reduced from 90 kg (198 lb) to 85 kg (187 lb) in one month. She had much more energy and was able to enjoy playing golf four times per week without difficulty, a feat she had not managed for at least 10 years previously.

Pre-diabetes

Although diabetes is obviously a very serious disease, what is not regularly recognised is the fact that 'pre-diabetes', the condition that precedes diabetes, is present in up to 24% of the population! This proportion obviously increases much higher in those over 50, and although they may not have overt diabetes, the symptoms and signs are usually developing for 10–15 years beforehand in a substantial proportion of the population.

And the most important sign of pre-diabetes is the measurement of the hormone insulin. Insulin is the classical marker for type 2 diabetes and increases before the blood sugar levels, so the measurement of insulin gives us a very accurate indication of the presence or absence of pre-diabetes. Consider this: as stated above, up to 24% of the population have pre-diabetes, which makes this one of the commonest conditions in the United Kingdom. It can lead to heart disease, eye disease, kidney disease and nerve disease – and it can be prevented by diet, exercise and reducing stress levels!

The following is an example of a patient who attended the clinic with gradually increasing weight over a period of 2–3 years, and the common symptoms of lethargy and visual problems. He was a 53-year-old banker with a weight of 99 kg (218 lb) and, although the blood sugar level was within normal limits of 5.6 mmol/l, the insulin level was 27.4 mmol/l (normal 5.0). In other words, his insulin level was more than five times normal! The patient was almost inevitably going to develop diabetes and undoubtedly the symptoms he was developing were indicative of the condition.

He adhered to the programme very conscientiously and within one month his weight had reduced by 5 kg (11 lb) to 94 kg (207 lb). The insulin level had reduced to 15.5 mmol/l and he was well on his way to recovery.

Within a further month his weight had reduced to 88 kg (194 lb), 11 kg (24 lb) less than two months previously, and his insulin level was 9.5, which is still above normal but had reduced by 60% in two months purely on the programme. He was effectively out of the danger zone for diabetes, and his insulin level has continued to reduce to normal levels subsequently.

In other words, because the diseases of ageing are occurring with age, it does not mean that you have to allow them to develop. A simple change in lifestyle can make a massive difference to the development of disease.

Cholesterol

CASE STUDY 1

John is the highly successful managing director of a major international company. He had recently had a cardiac event, having been noted on a recent examination to have narrowing of a coronary artery by 98%! The narrowing was obviously caused by stress and cholesterol plaques, and he required a stent to be introduced into the artery immediately as an emergency; a stent is a structure which mechanically opens the artery. He was on high-dose statins to reduce the cholesterol levels which were not successful in controlling the problem. His weight was 90 kg (198 lb). On commencing the programme:

- **Cholesterol level was 5.6 mmol/l**
- **HDL level of 1.3 mmol/l**
- **LDL level of 3.7 mmol/l**

HDL is the protective form of cholesterol and LDL is the type that does damage in the arteries. Within one month on the programme, his cholesterol level had reduced to 4.6; however, much more significantly, the LDL level had reduced to 2.9 and the HDL level had increased to 1.6.

This demonstrates an excellent example of how the total cholesterol in itself is not the important measurement. Total cholesterol is a balance of 'good' and 'bad' cholesterols. It is important to have a higher level of the protective good HDL level and a lower level of the LDL level. As you can see, the LDL reduced by approximately 25% and the HDL increased by 25% over a period of one month. In other words, although the total cholesterol reduced by 25%, the ultimate result was much better because that 25% reduction had been achieved at the expense of the bad cholesterol, not the good cholesterol. During that period of time, his weight had reduced from 90 kg (198 lb) to 84 kg (185 lb) and he had much higher energy levels.

We should add that one year later, his cholesterol had reduced to such a degree that he was no longer taking statins and his cardiologist had reduced him to yearly follow-ups, which effectively means there was no ongoing medical problem!

CASE STUDY 2

Christina was a 61-year-old lady who had noticed increasing weight over a period of two years by about 15 kg (33 lb). She was being treated with statins for raised cholesterol levels which had reached 6.2 mmol/l; however, her cholesterol level was continuing to increase despite treatment. She was obviously very concerned about the possibility of heart disease and commenced the programme accordingly. When she commenced, her weight was 90 kg (198 lb).

Within one month her cholesterol level had reduced from 6.2 mmol/l to 5.9 mmol/l, and by the second month it was 4.5 mmol/l. The LDL cholesterol (the bad cholesterol), had reduced from 3.8 to 2.3 mmol/l, which obviously accounted for the significant drop in her total cholesterol. She had been noted to be significantly pre-diabetic at the time with an insulin level of 66.5, which reduced to 22.4 within one month and has continued to reduce subsequently. In other words, this patient reduced her cholesterol level from 6.2 to 4.5 mmol/l (28%) within two months on the programme alone. As her cholesterol level was by that stage within normal limits, and the LDL was well below normal (less than 3 mmol/l), at that stage we were commencing to reduce the level of statins, and subsequently she has managed to discontinue them completely.

These case studies are only intended to demonstrate the effects of correcting nutrition, lowering stress levels and appropriate exercise on controlling major medical conditions. It is important to emphasise that this is not using drugs or medications, but merely an adaptation of lifestyle. It is equally not intending to suggest that the programme will be similarly effective for everyone, as we are all individuals with different forms of disease which may lead to specific conditions. However, it is important to emphasise that most individuals lead a lifestyle which predisposes them to heart disease, stroke, diabetes and arthritis. If we change that lifestyle, the risk of these conditions will substantially reduce, and, for those who already have the conditions, the control will be significantly improved.

8 The Age Revolution Programme

THE PROGRAMME CONSISTS of three separate components:

- ■ **Nutritional**
- ■ **Physical**
- ■ **Stress relief**

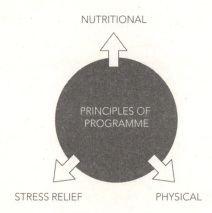

While each of these component parts has a major effect on health, the maximal benefit is gained by incorporating all three into a daily routine. In fact, the only effective way of achieving success is by establishing such a routine; without a definite commitment to physical exertion (however mild), stress relief and following a specific nutritional programme, on a daily basis, it simply will not happen as other 'important' issues will arise and take precedence. Remember, the aim of this exercise is to improve quality of life by slowing the ageing processes which would otherwise inevitably occur; it will only be effective if you commit to following the programme *on a daily basis.*

The following describes a 21-day programme to kick-start your journey. Each day includes a physical component and, most importantly, a winding-down exercise to relieve stress. Nutrition forms the basis of retarding the ageing process; you are, literally, what you eat, so adhere to the food plan. On this programme you will enjoy a wide range of delicious foods.

All you need is a little time and commitment to transform your future!

YOUR 21-DAY PROGRAMME

Day 1

Morning start

Stretching Exercises for Shoulders and Chest

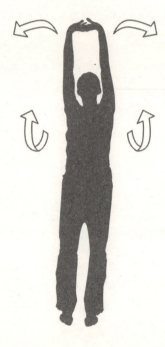

- Stand erect, feet approximately shoulder-width apart, and hands by your sides.

- Slowly raise the arms in a circular motion away from the body and above the head, keeping the arms straight at all times, until they just touch.

- Slowly lower the arms to the side.

- It may not be possible to raise the arms fully above the head initially, and do not strain excessively, so if you feel any tension stop at that point and lower the arms slowly to the sides.

■ Repeat this about 10 times for the first 10 days.

■ Gradually during that period try to raise the arms higher until they actually touch above your head but do not strain.

Menu plan

Breakfast: Halloumi kebabs and tomato (page 194) <u>or</u> porridge [page 166]

Lunch: Pumpkin and ginger soup [page 178]

Dinner: Smoked trout with watercress and mint sauce [page 186]

Winding down

Frankincense – blend in a bath oil for relaxation.

Mix the bath oil (page 261), add 5ml to the bath, lie back and relax.

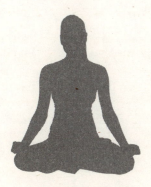

Day 2

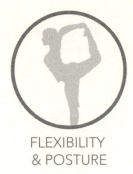

FLEXIBILITY
& POSTURE

Morning start

Hips and Thighs

■ Lie stretched out on the floor, arms by the sides.

■ Place the fitness ball under bent knees and relax.

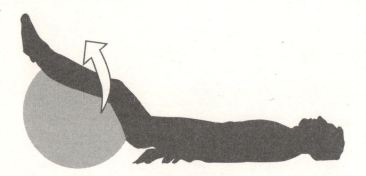

■ With arms outstretched, place the palms face down on the floor.

■ Gently pull your knees together and roll the fitness ball from side to side.

■ Perform this repetition about 5 times initially on each side for 2 weeks and gradually increase to 10 repetitions.

Menu plan

Breakfast: Poached eggs with tomato [page 167]

Lunch: Rocket and olive salad [page 218]

Dinner: Duck with mango purée [page 205]

Winding down

Promoting sleep with no stimulants – herbal tea.

Use a blend for insomnia (page 262) or just use 1 camomile teabag in a mug of hot water 1 hour before bedtime.

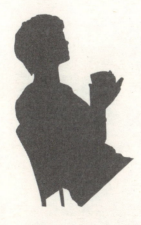

Day 3

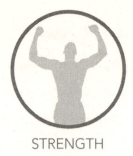

STRENGTH

Morning start

Chest and Bust Exercise

■ Sit erect with shoulders back and place hands together with elbows bent and arms horizontal approximately **15 cm (6 in)** from your chest.

■ Breathe in, press the palms together firmly and hold together for approximately **10 seconds** while holding your breath.

■ Release the pressure and relax for about **10 seconds**, then repeat this exercise **4 times**.

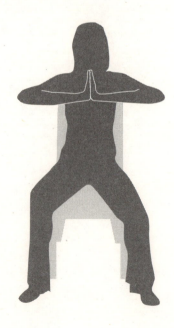

Menu plan

Breakfast: Oregano and tomato bagel [page 238]

Lunch: Lamb cutlets with garlic butter sauce [page 195]

Dinner: Tuna steaks with asparagus [page 189]

Winding down

A relaxing hand massage (page 262) with lavender oil.

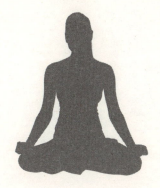

Day 4

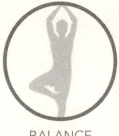

BALANCE

Morning start

Balance

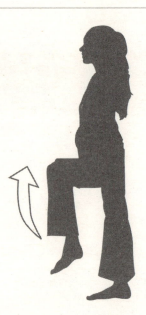

- This is best performed at the beginning of the day as it sets the tone for muscle balance throughout the day.

- Stand erect with both feet together looking straight ahead.

- Place your hands on hips.

- Slowly raise the left leg until the knee is level with the hip. If it is not possible to raise the leg to this height, do not worry, simply raise it a little and maintain your balance looking straight ahead for about 10 seconds.

- Balance on one foot.

- Try to point the foot downward during the exercise.

▓ Hold for a count of 10 and then slowly lower the leg to the ground.

▓ Repeat the exercise with the right leg.

▓ For the first week simply raise each leg off the ground on one occasion, but gradually build up to 5 repetitions to each leg per day after a period of about 2 weeks.

Menu plan

Breakfast: Breakfast platter [page 170]

Lunch: Smoked salmon frittata [page 184]

Dinner: Stir-fried vegetables [page 235]

Winding down

Facial massage

Relaxing herbal skin treatment with frankincense facial cream (pages 261 and 263).

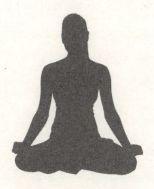

Day 5

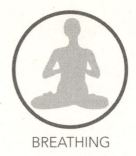

Morning start

HeartMath/Soothing Tea (Camomile)

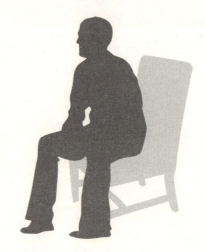

■ Ten-minute heart focus to stabilise your autonomic body rhythms and relieve stress at the start of the day (see page 59).

Menu plan

Breakfast: Fresh fruit with natural yoghurt [page 171]

Lunch: Halloumi and fennel salad [page 216]

Dinner: Spicy beef patties [page 198]

Winding down

Glass of organic wine with a relaxing oil in a burner.

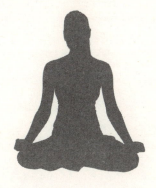

Day 6

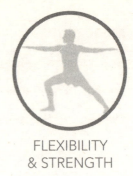

Morning start

The Upper Arms

▓ Stand erect, shoulders pulled back and head looking straight ahead.

▓ With arms held straight, clasp both hands behind your back.

▓ Slowly raise your arms behind your back as high as you can, but do not strain.

▓ Hold the contraction for about 3 seconds then release.

▓ Repeat this exercise on a further 4 occasions.

▓ Once again within a relatively short period of time you will feel the increased tone and tension in the upper back and upper arm muscles.

▓ After 4 weeks of this exercise increase the repetitions to 10 per day.

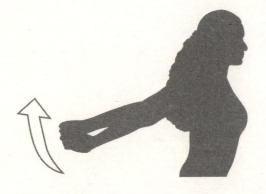

Menu plan

Breakfast: Traditional bacon and eggs

Lunch: Mushrooms with garlic [page 230]

Dinner: Chicken and pine nut salad [page 219]

Winding down

Try slippery elm to aid digestion after a heavy meal.

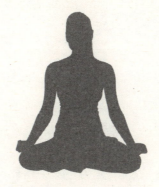

Day 7

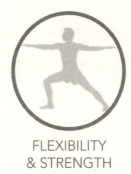

FLEXIBILITY
& STRENGTH

Morning start

Brisk Walk for 20 Minutes

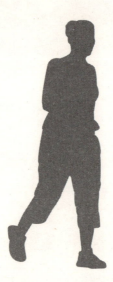

■ Take a brisk early morning walk for 20 minutes, essential for circulation and oxygenation of the tissues.

Menu plan

Breakfast: Omelette with a choice of filling [page 169]

Lunch: Tarragon chicken [page 204]

Dinner: Rocket and olive salad [page 218]

Winding down

Self massage for stress relief using arnica salve (page 264), massaging the salve gently over the affected joint(s).

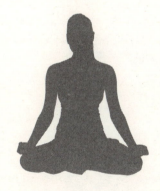

Day 8

Morning start

Upper Thighs and Bottom

■ Sit on the ground with your back against a wall, sitting erect.

■ Stretch your legs out straight in front, and then gradually pull them up towards you with the soles together.

■ If you cannot pull them completely together do not worry, even partially with be enough.

■ Place your hands on the ground beside you to balance, then gradually (slowly) rock from side to side, feeling the pressure on both the buttocks and the back of the thighs as you rock gently.

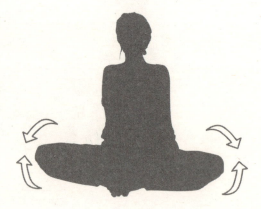

Menu plan

Breakfast: Porridge [page 166]

Lunch: Pumpkin and ginger soup [page 178]

Dinner: Chicken and pine nut salad [page 219]

Winding down

HeartMath (page 63) with soothing lemon balm tisane (page 262).

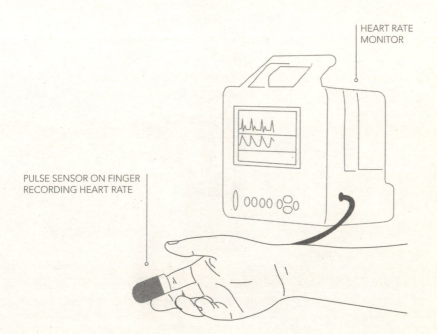

HEART RATE
MONITOR

PULSE SENSOR ON FINGER
RECORDING HEART RATE

Day 9

POSTURE

Morning start

Stretching Exercises for Shoulders and Chest

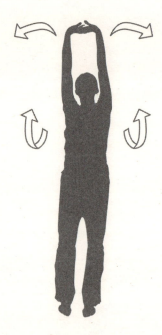

- Stand erect, feet approximately shoulder-width apart, and hands by your sides.

- Slowly raise the arms in a circular motion away from the body and above the head, keeping the arms straight at all times, until they just touch.

- Slowly lower the arms to the sides.

- It may not be possible to raise the arms fully above the head initially, and do not strain excessively, so if you feel any tension stop at that point and lower the arms slowly to the sides.

- Repeat this about 10 times.

- Gradually during that period try to raise the arms higher until they actually touch above your head but do not strain.

- After a further month, hold a small weight in each hand (which could be a soft drink bottle or a small tin) as this will increase the resistance and improve the exercise.

Menu plan

Breakfast: Two poached eggs with tomato [page 167]

Lunch: Stilton and toasted walnut pâté [page 214]

Dinner: Smoked trout with watercress and mint sauce [page 186]

Winding down

Camomile tea for relaxation at the end of the day.

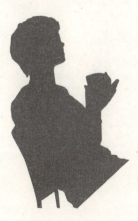

Day 10

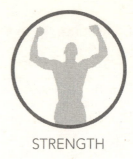

STRENGTH

Morning start

Strengthening Exercises for Upper Back

- Sit erect on a dining chair with the backrest at a distance of approximately 15 cm (6 in).
- Place both hands behind the back on either side of the chair and grasp the chair firmly.
- Take in a deep breath and press your hands together trying to compress the chair and hold the contraction for about 10 seconds.
- Release and rest for about 10 seconds and then repeat on a further 4 occasions.
- Once again, within a few days you will soon feel the improved tone and muscle power in your upper back from this simple exercise.

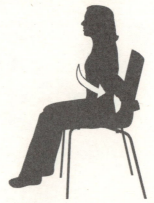

Menu plan

Breakfast: Toasted cheese with herbs [page 168]

Lunch: Aubergines with yoghurt and cucumber [page 217]

Dinner: Steak with salsa verde [page 196]

Winding down

Relaxing hand massage with orange oil. A great routine for a couple.

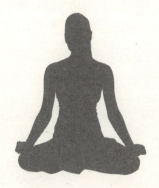

Day 11

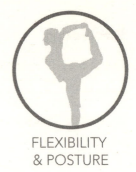

Morning start

Hips and Thighs

- Lie stretched out on the floor, arms by the sides.
- Place the fitness ball under bent knees and relax.
- With arms outstretched, place the palms face down on the floor.
- Gently pull your knees together and roll the fitness ball from side to side.
- Perform this repetition about 10 times on each side.

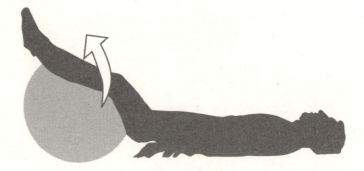

Menu plan

Breakfast: Strawberry and orange smoothie [page 175]

Lunch: Mussel soup with lime and coriander [page 181]

Dinner: Poached chicken with spring vegetables [page 208]

Winding down

Facial massage with rosehip seed oil (page 268).

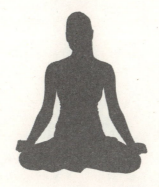

Day 12

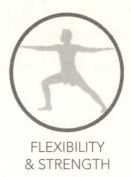

FLEXIBILITY
& STRENGTH

Morning start

Brisk 20-Minute Walk to Improve Circulation

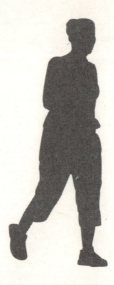

■ Take a brisk early morning walk for 20 minutes for mental relaxation as well as the more obvious physical attributes!

Menu plan

Breakfast: Warm hearty porridge [page 166]

Lunch: Rocket and olive salad [page 218]

Dinner: Duck with mango purée [page 205]

Winding down

Frankincense

Mix the bath oil (page 261), add 5 ml to the bath, lie back and relax.

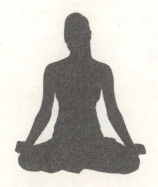

Day 13

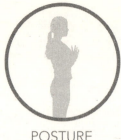

Morning start

Leg Stretching

- Stand in an open door frame with your back resting against the doorpost.

- Lift one leg and place the sole of the foot against the other doorpost at whatever height is convenient to you.

- Do not strain by trying to lift the leg too high.

- Take a deep breath and hold your breath, then press your leg firmly against the doorpost and keep the contraction for about 10 seconds.

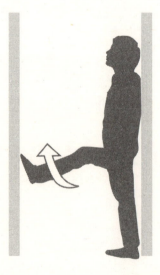

- Relax for about 10 seconds and then repeat for a further 4 times.

■ Allow a period of about **30** seconds to relax and then repeat the exercise with the other leg.

Menu plan

Breakfast: Avocado and toast [page 172]

Lunch: Courgette and basil soup [page 180]

Dinner: Pheasant with lemon butter and French beans [page 210]

Winding down

HeartMath (breathing) with soothing oil (of your choice) in a burner.

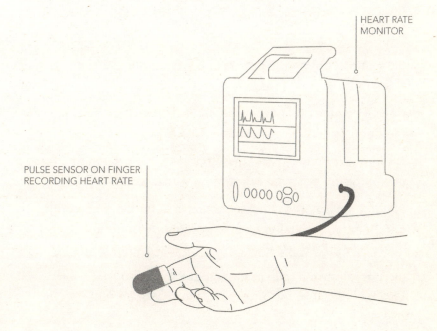

HEART RATE
MONITOR

PULSE SENSOR ON FINGER
RECORDING HEART RATE

Day 14

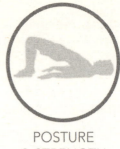

POSTURE
& STRENGTH

Morning start

Waistline

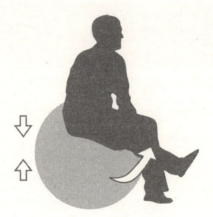

■ Sit comfortably on the fitness ball with hands on hips to the
side.

■ Gently bounce on the fitness ball 2–3 times then start to raise
the right leg off the ground and back down.

■ On the next bounce raise the left leg off the ground and back
down, raising each leg alternately with each bounce.

■ Initially have 10 repetitions of each side for the first month,
and then gradually increase the number of repetitions.

■ As you will see this is a very safe and simple exercise and
increases muscle tone in the upper thighs and waist very
easily.

Menu plan

Breakfast: Berry smoothie [page 174]

Lunch: Slow-cooked lamb and rosemary [page 197]

Dinner: Spicy whiting with courgette and parsley salad
[page 188]

Winding down

*Glass of organic wine with soothing music in the
background.*

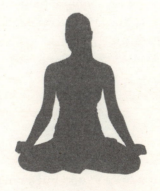

Day 15

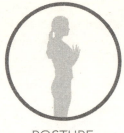
Morning start

Upper Back Exercise

■ Stand erect, shoulders back and arms by the sides.

■ Raise your arms to be level with the shoulders with fingers touching together held horizontally.

■ Keep arms horizontal at shoulder height and pull the elbows back as far as they can, feeling the tension in the upper back.

■ Gradually release the tension in the upper back and allow the shoulders to move forward to the resting position, and then repeat a further 10 times.

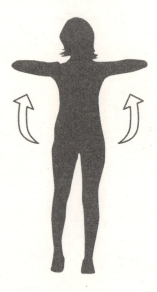

■ Continue this routine for 2 weeks, and then gradually increase to 15 repetitions per day.

Menu plan

Breakfast: Breakfast platter [page 170]

Lunch: Stilton and toasted walnut pâté [page 214]

Dinner: Salmon steak parcels [page 187]

Winding down

Self-massage stress release with ginger salve (page 265), gently massaging salve into aching joints.

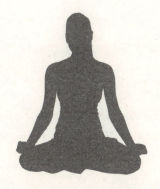

Day 16

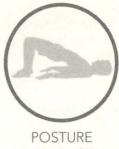

Morning start

Abdomen and Tummy

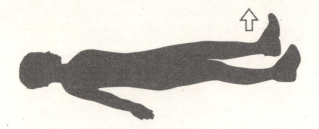

- Lie flat on the floor with arms outstretched.

- Very slowly, keeping the leg straight, lift one leg off the floor about 1–2 inches (2.5–5 cm), and hold for 2–3 seconds, then slowly lower the leg to the floor.

- Repeat the exercise with the other leg, again holding the leg off the floor for about 2–3 seconds then slowly lowering to the floor.

- Repeat this exercise with both legs separately about 5 times for the first 4 weeks, then gradually increase to 10 repetitions.

Menu plan

Breakfast: Fresh fruit with natural yoghurt [page 171]

Lunch: Oat-crusted cod [page 185]

Dinner: Stir-fried vegetables [page 235]

Winding down

Promoting sleep, no stimulants – camomile tea.

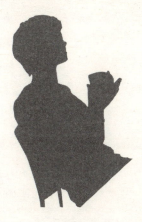

Day 17

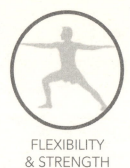

FLEXIBILITY
& STRENGTH

Morning start

Neck Exercises

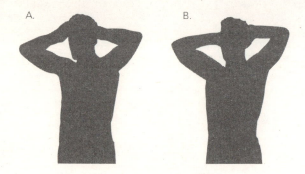

A.   B.

- ▨ Take in a deep breath and hold.

- ▨ Place both hands on the front of the forehead, and press your head forward against the fixed hands as firmly as you can.

- ▨ Hold for 10 seconds and release.

- ▨ To balance the muscles at the back of the neck, place your hands behind your head, take in a deep breath, and press the head back against the hands holding firmly for about 10 seconds.

- ▨ Relax and breathe normally.

Menu plan

Breakfast: Oregano and tomato bagel [page 238]

Lunch: Smoked salmon frittata [page 184]

Dinner: Chicken paprika [page 202]

Winding down

A relaxing hand massage with ginger salve (page 265).

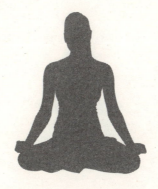

Day 18

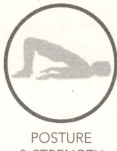

Morning start

Tension Release

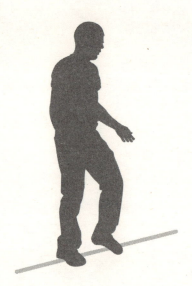

- Place a thin, straight smooth stick or broom handle on the floor.

- Standing erect, place one foot on the broom handle then the other, resting both feet on the stick in an erect position.

- Gradually lift the right foot onto ball of the foot, transferring weight to the left then slowly lower the right foot onto the stick and lift the left foot onto the ball, moving away from the stick.

- Gradually, in a stepwise manner, repeat this exercise about 10 times, and then step off the stick carefully.

■ This exercise should be performed slowly as it gradually releases muscle tension from the feet, and therefore throughout the whole body.

Menu plan

Breakfast: Poached eggs [page 167]

Lunch: Tarragon chicken [page 204]

Dinner: Spicy whiting with courgette and parsley salad [page 188]

Winding down

Promoting circulation with prickly ash tincture (page 266).

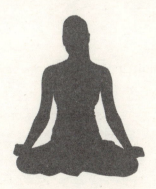

Day 19

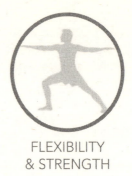

FLEXIBILITY
& STRENGTH

Morning start

Brisk 20-Minute Walk

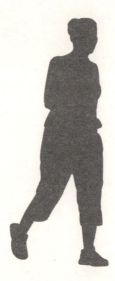

▨ Walking for 20 minutes three times per week is proven to increase circulation and cardiac health.

Menu plan

Breakfast: Strawberry and orange smoothie [page 175]

Lunch: Lamb cutlets with garlic butter sauce [page 195]

Dinner: Stir-fried vegetables [page 235]

Winding down

Relaxing bath with soothing frankincense and lavender oil (page 261).

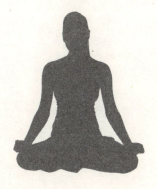

Day 20

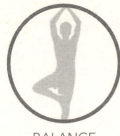

BALANCE

Morning start

Balance

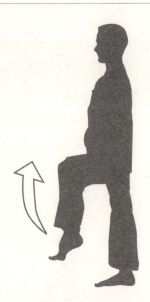

- This is best performed at the beginning of the day as it sets the tone for muscle balance throughout the day.

- Stand erect with both feet together looking straight ahead.

- Place hands on hips.

- Slowly raise the left leg until the knee is level with the hip. If it is not possible to raise the leg to this height, do not worry, simply raise it a little and maintain your balance looking straight ahead for about 10 seconds.

- Balance on one foot.

- Try to point the foot downward during the exercise.

■ Hold for a count of 10 and then slowly lower the leg to the ground.

■ Repeat the exercise with the right leg.

■ Perform 5 repetitions with each leg.

Menu plan

Breakfast: Omelette with filling [page 169]

Lunch: Halloumi and fennel salad [page 216]

Dinner: Smoked trout with watercress and mint sauce [page 186]

Winding down

Relaxing facial massage with frankincense facial cream (page 261).

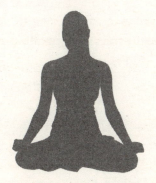

Day 21

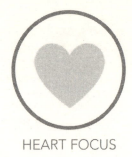

Morning start

HeartMath/Soothing Herbal Tea

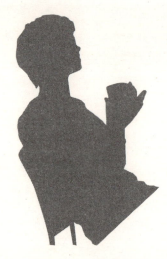

- Stress hormones are released during sleep so you can actually awaken with stress. Controlling cardiac rhythms has a calming effect on the approach to the day.

- And complete the process of relaxation with a soothing camomile tea.

Menu plan

Breakfast: Traditional bacon and eggs

Lunch: Slow-cooked lamb and rosemary [page 197]

Dinner: Spicy beef patties [page 198]

Winding down

A glass of organic wine and a relaxing oil (of your choice) in a burner.

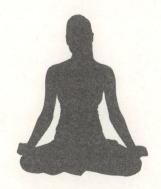

9 Nutrition for health – a practical guide

FIRSTLY YOU NEED to understand and appreciate the importance of food preparation. It is incredibly easy to lapse into the same old routine. This is the time to rekindle your interest in *real* food, or to establish an interest in health. Food is important! It provides us with all of the essential nutrients that we need for health and essentially balances the body's nutritional status. Of course, our bodies can cope with the consumption of unhealthy foods for a certain period of time, but, as we all know, in the long run this causes a silent form of damage which ultimately becomes overt with the development of:

■ **Diabetes**
■ **Heart disease**
■ **Hypertension**
■ **Arthritis**
■ **Obesity**
■ **Osteoporosis**

But these diseases are not inevitable, they are in the majority of cases caused by lifestyle. And amazingly you can actually prevent most of these by the simple expedient of a healthy lifestyle!

There are essentially two types of individual: those who are genuinely interested in food and those for whom food is a mere expedient. We need to rekindle interest in cooking in those who are competent and engender it in those who are not. The aim is not to create Michelin chefs, but rather to increase people's culinary proficiency so that they may derive greater enjoyment from the techniques of food preparation.

Because not only will rekindling an interest in food improve the quality of life as you age, it also has major psychological effects. Cooking is a major form of reducing stress and therefore reducing the autonomic effects on the body. When you cook for yourself and perhaps a partner (unlike preparing food for a large family, which is obviously stressful) you are inevitably:

- **distracted from other negative thoughts**
- **reconnecting with your senses with the various aromas, colours, tastes, textures and even sounds of food.**

Virtually everyone enjoys food. Many think it is enjoyable just to eat pre-prepared food or at restaurants because it is easier, and that is a perfectly reasonable view, but if you actually take an interest in preparing your own food, with natural ingredients, not only will you be healthier, but you will achieve a higher level of personal satisfaction – which, in turn, will inevitably reduce stress levels.

As individuals, we create a particular style for ourselves in many aspects of our daily life: fashion choices, career choices and, of course, lifestyle choices. So why not eating choices? Simply because cooking is considered a partially menial activity, it does not mean it needs to be so!

By developing your own nutritional plan through Nutritional Coherence, you will start to take control of your own health. Obviously, it would be absurd to suggest that Nutritional Coherence can prevent all forms of disease and debility; nevertheless, you can make substantial positive changes to your health by relatively simple lifestyle and nutritional adaptations. In those over 40, nutrient absorption can decline and therefore it is important to maintain a high level of nutrition. The body's stores of vitamins and minerals which are particularly reduced at this time of life are vitamin B6, vitamin D and zinc. Zinc-rich foods, which are particularly important for the immune system, include shellfish, pumpkin seeds and lean meat. Vitamin B6 is common in turkey, fish, peppers, and green vegetables such as Brussels sprouts and watercress. Vitamin D is most readily obtained from oily fish such as mackerel, herring, tuna, salmon and sardines. Although there is a certain amount of vitamin D in daily foods, the highest levels are undoubtedly in oily fish. It is important to understand that there about 15 vitamins and 15 minerals which are known to be needed in small amounts for health; however, what you should realise is apart from vitamins D and K they are only available from food and therefore it is absolutely essential to obtain the necessary nutrition either from food or from supplements, although obviously fresh food is best.

We all lead very structured and organised lifestyles. It can be daunting to consider changing, but you will undoubtedly reap the benefits if you do.

Of course, *how* to prepare food is just as important as *what* to prepare. There is no point in providing a nutritious variety of foods with healthy ingredients which are ruined by preparation and cooking. And while this may seem obvious, it really is not. For example, boiling vegetables is an excellent method of removing all of the nutrition from them into the water, whereas stir-frying retains virtually all of the nutrients within the vegetables. Simple as that! It is very easy to prepare quick, nutritious and delicious meals, from healthy ingredients, by following a few rules. In this way, anyone can cook well and enjoy a very healthy and nutritious lifestyle.

We have divided the various food groups into:

- **Beef, pork and lamb**
- **Poultry**
- **Fish and shellfish**
- **Vegetables**
- **Herbs and spices**

To make it simple, each section is subdivided into:

- **What to buy, and**
- **Cooking methods**

Beef, pork and lamb

What to buy

All these are obviously purchased either fresh or frozen, and with the fresh you have the option of freezing and using at a later date.

Cooking methods

▪ Ready-cooked

Ready-cooked meats are the ideal solution for anyone wishing a fast diet which is also very healthy. It is also the perfect solution for anyone who can't cook and does not want to learn. All forms of cold sliced meats are equally healthy and are packed with nutrition. For example salamis, hams, pastrami, chorizo, pepperoni ... the list is almost endless. And, of course, there are the simple varieties such as sliced roast beef, roast pork and roast ham.

▪ Frying

'Frying' refers to either stir-frying or shallow frying in a little extra-virgin olive oil. Deep fat frying is never healthy and should not be used.

On the contrary, stir-frying or light frying is not unhealthy. Extra-virgin olive oil contains omega 3 fatty acids, and the oils allow fat-soluble vitamins (A, D, E and K) to be absorbed from food. If there is no fat in the diet, fat-soluble vitamins cannot be absorbed and this is a common cause of vitamin D deficiency leading to osteoporosis.

The advantage of stir-frying meat products is that the meat is cooked very quickly and retains much of its nutrition and vitamins. The easiest way of cooking meat quickly and healthily is to slice the meat finely and cook in a matter of 3–4 minutes, thereby retaining all of its healthy nutrients.

▪ Grilling

Grilling is a very simple method of cooking larger cuts of meat such as chops and steaks and retaining most of the healthy nutrients.

For example, a medium steak will take between 5–8 minutes (turning once) and requires very little supervision.

Baking

It is important to realise that cheaper cuts of steak (or any meat), such as those used in casseroles, have exactly the same nutrition as the more expensive cuts. So casserole meat is as healthy as the finest fillet steak. The only difference is that it takes longer to cook, but, of course, the actual *preparation time* for the meal is exactly the same as if it was a finer cut. The only difference is that you have to prepare ahead because the casserole takes about two hours to cook.

Roasting

Roasting takes longer than simply frying or grilling, but it really only involves a little forethought and preparation rather than any extra time. How simple can it be to place a joint of beef, lamb or pork in the oven with some tasty herbs and enjoy a delicious meal about two hours later? It does not get much simpler.

Microwave

Cooking meat in a microwave is another speedy option. There is little preparation time, the meat cooks in a relatively short time, and equally importantly, it shrinks much less than in a conventional oven.

Poultry

What to buy

Poultry can be purchased fresh or frozen, and fresh is definitely best. Although that does not mean that it cannot be ready-prepared and ready to eat, as chicken breasts, thighs, wings and drumsticks can just as easily be purchased freshly cooked.

Cooking methods

▓ Ready-cooked

Poultry is probably the most readily available of the precooked meat varieties. It can be purchased as ready-cooked drumsticks, wings, thighs and breasts, and is available in many varieties with different sauces which are relatively healthy. Turkey and chicken breast can be purchased as sliced and cooked cold meats and so this type of food is available to everyone.

▓ Stir-frying

Once again, poultry is particularly suitable for fast and nutritious meals, even for those who can't cook. Chicken or turkey breasts sliced into strips and stir-fried in extra-virgin olive oil, with some sliced vegetables (such as peppers and spring onions), fresh ginger or garlic and a little soy sauce provide a quick, delicious and nutritious meal in minutes.

▓ Frying

Turkey and chicken breasts can be shallow-fried in two tablespoons of extra-virgin olive oil. Deep fat frying, which is commonly associated with chicken, is not healthy and should not be used. And never forget turkey mince, which is even more delicious than its meat counterpart and is easily browned with a Bolognese sauce to provide a very healthy meal.

▓ Baking

Baking chicken, duck or pheasant is a simple and delicious way of cooking. Place the segments (breast, drumsticks, wings or thighs) on a greased baking tray and cook for 30 minutes in a preheated oven. It really could not be much simpler!

▓ Microwave

Similar to meat, poultry segments cook quickly and safely in a microwave oven. Shrinkage is less than in a conventional oven, and if not overcooked, the texture remains moist and tender.

■ **Roasting**

Poultry is ideal for roasting, with the advantage of requiring relatively little preparation time.

Fish and shellfish

What to buy

Fish and shellfish are always better fresh, in terms of taste. However, this type of food has the advantage of being readily available either tinned or frozen and is equally nutritious. Particularly as we age, it really is important to include oily fish (herring, mackerel, sardines, tuna and salmon) at least twice a week as they contain the essential omega 3 fatty acids and are the highest source of vitamin D and calcium in the diet, deficiency of which is the cause of osteoporosis.

Cooking methods

■ **Ready-cooked**

The variety of pre-cooked fish and shellfish available is almost unlimited. It is important to realise that all of these provide just as many of the essential vitamins and minerals as the fresh variety, even if perhaps they are not quite as tasty. Pre-cooked fish (such as kippers, mackerel and smoked salmon) or tinned (tuna, salmon, mackerel, sardines and herring) are delicious, healthy meals that are readily available. Shellfish (such as prawns or crab) are available freshly cooked and can be easily combined with vegetables or sauces to provide an instant healthy meal.

Of course, frozen fish (salmon, haddock, cod) and shellfish (scallops, prawns, cockles and mussels) are also readily available and after quickly defrosting can cook in just a few minutes. Once again, these varieties are almost as healthy as their fresh counterparts.

▓ Stir-frying

Fresh fish is easily fried with a little extra-virgin olive oil and is ready in less than 5 minutes – the natural fast food!

▓ Baking

Similarly, fish is ideally suited to baking as it cooks perfectly within about 15–20 minutes.

▓ Steaming

Steaming is healthy for almost every type of food. It retains all the vitamins and minerals and is ready very quickly.

▓ Grilling

You really have to watch fish if you intend to grill it as it can dry out very quickly. Shellfish are certainly not suitable for grilling.

▓ Microwave

Once again, microwave cooking is very suitable for this type of food and cooks fish and shellfish very quickly, maintaining their tenderness and essential nutrients.

Vegetables

What to buy

Once again, fresh is best! There really is no comparison between fresh vegetables and tinned or frozen varieties. And don't forget fresh herbs! These are widely available and the antioxidant properties of herbs are rivalled only by those of spices.

Cooking methods

▓ Ready-prepared

You can technically buy ready-cooked vegetables, such as tinned or frozen, but these are really not very good, either in taste or in health qualities.

On the other hand *ready-prepared* vegetables are available widely. Mangetout, broccoli, French beans, sugar snap peas and bean sprouts are just a few of the varieties available for instant use.

Stir-frying

Stir-frying is a wonderful way of cooking vegetables. They retain almost all of their natural healthy ingredients because they are cooked very quickly, and all you need to do is slice them finely to ensure rapid cooking.

Steaming

Steaming is a healthy method of cooking for virtually everything, but particularly for vegetables as they lose virtually none of their nutrition and effectively retain all of the flavour.

Microwave

Once again, cooking vegetables in a microwave oven is healthy and quick and retains most of the healthy nutrients.

The only method of cooking vegetables to be avoided at all costs is 'boiling'! Essentially, when the vegetables are chopped up and boiled for some time, almost all of the essential nutrients are lost into the surrounding water, as is the flavour!

Herbs and spices

The first question, of course, is exactly what are herbs? Herbs are plants or parts of plants such as the fruits, flowers and leaves, which can be used in a variety of ways, but the main applications are:

- **Medicinal use, such as camomile which is used to promote relaxation**
- **Therapeutic use, such as in essential oils for massages or aromatic baths**
- **Culinary use.**

Of course, it is immediately apparent that the plants' use in one sense cannot be separated from the other. In other words, if you can use a plant to flavour food advantageously, then it will inevitably have a medicinal purpose at the same time. And plants have been used medicinally for many thousands of years. Most of our current drugs originate from plant sources, so this is hardly surprising.

Spices, on the other hand, are usually regarded as the harder parts of aromatic plants. They include flora buds (cloves), dry fruits (cardamom), seeds (pepper), roots and stems (ginger) and even bark (cinnamon).

On a more practical level, herbs tend to be milder tasting, whereas spices tend to be stronger and are usually used in the dried form. However, there is a significant overlap between them and there are no hard and fast rules on the subject. The only common denominator is the fact that they are incredibly healthy with a high concentration of antioxidants, and have the capacity to make food taste wonderful.

Herbs and spices are an essential accompaniment to your diet, not just for the flavour that they impart to food but also for their significant medicinal advantages. In fact, if antioxidants are the key to preventing ageing, then herbs and spices are the key to providing antioxidants as they are the highest source of antioxidants in our diet. In other words, these simple and apparently nondescript additions to our food have actually the highest potential to prevent ageing of any substance known to man!

Herbs have been used for culinary and medicinal purposes for thousands of years. However, spices have had even more diverse uses such as infusions and poultices (fennel and aniseed), incense (liquorice, cloves and cinnamon), dyes such as turmeric, cosmetics (sesame seeds and myrrh), and even added to bath oils (saffron and ginger).

We have seen that there is an intense Nutritional Coherence in all these foods as they can be used for so many diverse purposes, all of which are healthy. But, of course, the aspect in which we are particularly interested is the prevention of ageing, and in this regard herbs and spices have immense properties as antioxidants. So it is definitely important that you keep a good supply of fresh and dried herbs and spices at all times and add them to your food appropriately. Herbs and spices don't deposit fat and can easily be added to enhance virtually any recipe and so they improve both health and flavour at the same time.

If you become adept at using herbs regularly, they will be incorporated into meals every day and so fresh herbs will never be wasted. It is very simple to grow them either in your garden or on a windowsill, but also important to keep a good supply of dried herbs constantly available. Similarly, a constant supply of spices is absolutely essential to promote health.

Of course, the most important aspect is how to use herbs and spices appropriately to achieve the maximum advantage – and the maximum flavour.

Herbs

We have appended a brief list of the most common herbs and spices used in cooking, and their favourite accompaniments to give you a few ideas.

BASIL

Basil is the 'king' of the herbs and in fact the name means 'king'. There are several types of basil plant; however, it is sweet basil that is mostly used in cooking. It is particularly appropriate to tomato, egg, mushroom and pasta dishes but it does have a rather strong flavour so use sparingly at the beginning until you become accustomed to it.

CORIANDER

Coriander can be used in many different ways: as fresh leaves, coriander seeds and, of course, ground coriander. Roots, stems and leaves can all be used but each has a different purpose. The roots tend to be used in curry pastes, the stems for increasing coriander flavour, and the leaves at the end of cooking as they can lose their flavour very quickly, as a garnish and as a flavouring.

Fresh coriander leaves are particularly appropriate to many different types of dishes. They are delicious with chicken, fish, curry, tomato and Thai dishes. Of course, ground coriander is used as an essential ingredient in curries and you can use whole coriander seeds with vegetables such as celery, beetroot and cauliflower.

DILL

Dill is a very fragrant plant with fine blue-green leaves. Its gentle feathery leaves impart a strong aniseed flavour, commonly used in Northern European dishes such as gravadlax, and also particularly appropriate with chicken and cream sauces. It is particularly suited to fish, and can also be added to green salads with cucumber, tomato salads, sour cream or avocados. It is an excellent accompaniment to omelettes, tomato and chicken soup.

It should be chopped and added at the end of cooking as it quickly loses its flavour.

PARSLEY

Parsley is probably the commonest and most widely used herb. There are several different varieties, including flat-leaf parsley and the commoner curly parsley. It is a herb which has health-giving properties such as the prevention of various types of anaemia, both iron-deficiency and pernicious anaemia; for example, 25 g of parsley provides more iron than 200 g of pork. In addition to iron, parsley has a high concentration of folate.

Apart from these very healthy attributes, parsley also has:

- **High concentration of calcium**
- **High concentration of antioxidants, particularly vitamin C and carotenes.**

This humble herb also has very potent diuretic qualities: just 25 g of fresh parsley, of whatever variety, stimulates kidney function.

The uses of parsley are ubiquitous: green salads, sauces, vegetables and soups, with white sauce and fish. Parsley is frequently added to dishes which contain garlic, as it is known to slightly soften the flavour.

COMFREY

Comfrey has large and rough green leaves, which need to be chopped for cooking. It is particularly useful cooked on its own with plain green vegetables such as spinach or watercress. It is frequently added to white sauce with fish, or to green salads.

TARRAGON

Tarragon leaves are narrow and shiny and it has greenish-white flowers. The herb has ubiquitous applications and is particularly useful for roast dishes such as meat, poultry and fish. It can be added to French dressing, and the leaves give an additional flavour to green salads. Like parsley, it is a particularly suitable accompaniment to white sauce. With a hint of aniseed in its flavouring, it is a common accompaniment to many classic French dishes. When used in flavouring vinegar and sauces for poultry, it is essential to have French tarragon and not the Russian variety, which has a more bitter flavour.

HORSERADISH

Horseradish is another herb with large leaves. Its primary use is as a condiment, when grated into cream. As such it is a wonderful accompaniment to roast meats, especially beef. A lesser-known fact is that it aids the digestion of oily fish, such as mackerel or herring.

WATERCRESS

Watercress has the characteristic small rounded leaves which are commonly found in our freshwater streams. As with most herbs, it has integral health attributes:

■ **High levels of vitamins C and E and carotenes which are major antioxidants with the potential to prevent disease – and ageing.**

▪ Rich in folate and iron, which are essential to prevent both iron deficiency and pernicious anaemia.

▪ High concentrations of zinc, necessary for the function of the immune system.

▪ Good source of calcium, to help prevent osteoporosis.

It can be used in salads, although watercress soup is absolutely delicious.

LEMON THYME

Not surprisingly, the small green leaves are sweetly scented of lemon. Particularly useful in baked custard, salads and fruit desserts, it is also useful to add some sprigs when roasting a chicken.

MARJORAM

There are several forms of marjoram but by far the best for cooking is sweet marjoram. It is excellent with veal, chicken, lamb, pork, fish, tomatoes, vegetables and cheese dishes. Often added to olive oil dressings to spice them up, marjoram is delicious if added to vegetables such as squash and courgettes.

ROSEMARY

The green leaves are short and narrow and have the appearance of pine needles. It is commonly associated with roast lamb but can also be successfully added to fish dishes. Try halibut and rosemary for something different. It can also be added to fruit salads or egg dishes.

SAGE

Sage leaves tend to be large and soft. They are commonly added to roast pork but are also delicious with poultry dishes such as duck, or even with meat casseroles. Sage can be added to green salads, and gives a wonderful flavour to tomato-based meals.

THYME

Thyme is a rather woody herb and therefore you have to separate the tiny leaves from the stalks. It has a strong flavour and should be added sparingly to dishes such as meat and fish, casseroles and sauces. It imparts a wonderful flavour when added to vegetables like carrots or squash. There are many different varieties of thyme; however, it has the distinction of not losing its flavour during cooking and therefore is particularly appropriate for slow-cooked dishes.

BAY LEAVES

Particularly useful when poaching fish, or with venison casseroles. Very commonly added to curries or to meat and vegetable dishes – but remember to remove before serving!

FENNEL

A herb originating in the Mediterranean, fennel is easily grown in the UK climate. Growing up to 5 feet (1.5 m) tall, it is a very distinctive herb and has an equally distinctive aniseed flavour. Healthy properties include high levels of potassium and oestrogen effects with the application of improving menopausal symptoms.

It is a particularly suitable accompaniment to fish; fennel seeds are often added to breads and biscuits. The Florence variety has swollen stalk bases which we recognise as the vegetable.

CHIVES

Because of their ancestry, chives have an onion flavour and therefore can complement many dishes. They can be added to salads and soups of both meat and vegetable varieties. Chives can be blended with butter as a sauce for baked fish such as salmon and trout or even in egg dishes like omelettes.

GARLIC

Garlic is a ubiquitous addition to many different recipes. The bulb is chopped or grated, with a strong aroma, so must be used sparingly. Usually one clove is sufficient to bring out the necessary flavour in a savoury dish. It is often used in meat casseroles, soups and vegetable dishes, although any form of pasta dish is also particularly enhanced by garlic. Its strong flavour goes very well with meat, game and fish dishes.

CHERVIL

Chervil has fern-like, delicate leaves. The flavours of chervil disappear very quickly and it should only be added to dishes immediately before serving. A classic ingredient in béarnaise source, it has a hint of aniseed and is an outstandingly good accompaniment with fish.

Chervil is particularly tasty in a soup of its own name, although it can be added to butter sauces with vegetables or with egg and cheese dishes. It acts very well as a garnish over meat dishes such as beef and pork.

These are the commonest herbs used in cooking. The ways in which they can be prepared and used are almost unlimited: here is a small selection of techniques to demonstrate this.

How to chop herbs

This method can be used for most herbs and is best applied using a large heavy-bladed knife. Make sure the herbs are dry before chopping or they will form wet clumps, which are certainly not aesthetic.

- **Firstly chop off the stems, then form the leaves into a mound.**
- **With your non-dominant hand, carefully push the leaves under the knife while rapidly moving the knife up and down through the leaves. The easiest way is to press the tip of the**

knife against the cutting board, which helps to stabilise the knife and also prevents you from adding any fingers into the chopped herbs!

How to produce fennel shavings

Fennel shavings are best produced using a vegetable slicer set on the thinnest setting.

- Slide the fennel backwards and forwards over the blade, keeping your palm flat and your fingers spread to ensure that you don't get caught by the blade.
- Always use the hand guard when you get closer to the blade.

Chopping basil into chiffonade

This method is particularly useful for basil, but can actually be applied to any leafy green vegetable. Basil leaves turn black when chopped, so it is necessary to sprinkle a few drops of olive oil over the leaves and make sure they are thoroughly coated before chopping.

- Put the leaves into small piles of about 3 each and roll into a cylinder.
- Slice the leaves lengthways into thin strips to achieve the desired effect.
- For other green leaves such as chard and spinach (which do not turn black when chopped), sprinkling with olive oil is not necessary.

How to make a bouquet garni

Bouquet garni is a bundle of herbs that is often added to soups and casseroles to enhance the flavour. The classic French bouquet garni contains thyme, bay leaves and parsley stems. However, it is important to realise that the recipe for bouquet garni is not set in stone and tends to be dependent on the tastes of each individual country. For example, North Americans tend to tie the herbs in a package of cheese cloth, while in the south of France dried orange peel is often added.

Removing stems from salad herbs

It is important to remember that the small stems of most salad herbs are actually edible and impart a great deal of flavour to the meal, as in the use of parsley stems in bouquet garni, so don't try to remove all of the stems from such herbs. For example, with watercress, only remove the lower half of the stems, leaving the edible part intact.

How to make a hot vinaigrette

Hot vinaigrette utilises oil instead of butter which is a basic ingredient in a pan sauce, as the oil does not emulsify into the pan. This is because olive oil is not an emulsion and so it remains a separate liquid, whereas butter is an emulsion, emulsifies easily, and glazes the liquid. To produce a hot vinaigrette:

- Add some wine vinegar to a sauté pan to deglaze.
- Stir in one to two tablespoons of extra-virgin olive oil which completes the vinaigrette, then drizzle over the sautéed meal.

How to make an infused oil with basil

- Add two or three tablespoons of chopped basil leaves to a blender.
- Stir in one tablespoon of extra-virgin olive oil.
- Blend for about one minute.
- Transfer the mixture to a mixing bowl.
- Stir in three to four tablespoons of extra-virgin olive oil, cover and leave to infuse at room temperature for about 12 hours.
- Strain the oil through a fine sieve.
- Transfer to glass bottles and store at room temperature.
- This should keep for about one month.

How to make a herb butter

Herb butter is particularly useful to have on hand as it can transform the simplest meal into a delicacy, such as grilled fish, shellfish, meat or even vegetables. Tarragon butter is one of the commonest but it can be made with most herbs.

- **Soften the butter initially by kneading slightly.**
- **Add the butter to a blender with one tablespoon of fresh tarragon leaves and blend together.**
- **To serve the butter as discs (which is the easiest way with grilled meats and vegetables) place the butter on a sheet of greaseproof paper, roll the butter within the paper into a sausage shape, and twist the ends of the greaseproof paper to seal.**
- **Set aside in the fridge for 1–2 hours.**
- **It is then relatively simple to slice the flavoured butter into even rounds.**

How to make a pesto sauce

The basic pesto sauce recipe incorporates basil, garlic, parmesan cheese and olive oil.

For two

2 tbsp fresh basil leaves, chopped
1 garlic clove, peeled and chopped
25 g freshly grated Parmesan cheese
30 ml extra-virgin olive oil

- **Add the basil, garlic and Parmesan to a blender and chop for about one minute.**
- **Blend in the extra-virgin olive oil slowly to achieve a smooth and even consistency.**

Of course this basic recipe is amended according to taste and geographical location: for example, the French pistou contains tomatoes; the more traditional Ligurian recipes would add pine nuts.

Now it is important that we look at spices that can also be added to enhance health.

Spices

Spices have the distinction of being the food with the highest quantities of antioxidants per unit volume. In other words, they have a very high concentration of antioxidants indeed, and are the ideal food to prevent free radical formation and therefore prevent ageing. Add spices appropriately and sparingly to your food for wonderful added flavours and excellent health-giving properties. We will describe some of the commonest of the spices, although the list is very large indeed.

CAYENNE

Cayenne is a capsicum; however, it is related to chillies rather than to peppers. A highly spiced food, which is commonly added to curries and savouries such as pastes.

PAPRIKA

Paprika is another capsicum or sweet pepper. Originating in Hungary, it is still used today to flavour many of the nation's dishes, particularly goulash.

CHILLIES

Another member of the capsicum family, obviously a ubiquitous plant, chillies originate from South America and Mexico. Be careful, the hottest chillies are the smaller ones, particularly the small red chillies. Obvious uses of chillies are to spice up any hot dish such as curry.

CINNAMON

Cinnamon is the rolled inner bark of a tree which grows in India and Sri Lanka. Its commonest use now is as a flavouring for sweet dishes such as cakes and mulled wine, although it can be added to meat and fish dishes.

SAFFRON

Saffron is the most expensive of the spices, being made from the stigmas of a species of crocus, the saffron crocus. It is particularly used in Italian risottos, Spanish paellas and fish soups – but use sparingly!

TURMERIC

Ground turmeric is a common ingredient in curries (and the European curry powders), relishes such as piccalilli, and mustard. It provides the distinctive colour of these dishes.

CUMIN

With turmeric and coriander, cumin powder forms the base of many curries. It is common in spice mixtures such as curry powder and garam masala. Cumin goes very well with vegetable and fish dishes and even with pulses.

LEMONGRASS

Lemongrass is probably the most characteristic flavouring of dishes from Southeast Asia, particularly Thailand. It is used as a whole dry stalk to flavour the dish, then discarded before the dish is served. It goes well with coconut milk and most forms of Thai cuisine.

CARDAMOM

Cardamom comes primarily as seeds rather than powder and is one of the main ingredients in curry powder and garam masala and is even added to coffee in the Middle East.

CLOVES

Cloves are actually immature flower buds. Although originally regarded as black peppercorns (which were a luxury several centuries ago), they are now commonly used in both savoury and sweet dishes, and particularly in drinks such as mulled wine. In India they are incorporated into meat and rice dishes, and as one of the main ingredients of garam masala.

FENNEL SEEDS

These are commonly used in Indian cookery in recipes of meat, fish and vegetables and even in Europe in a salami from Florence.

STAR ANISE

There is no mistaking this particular spice as it is shaped as a star. Even more characteristically, it has a strong smell of aniseed and liquorice. It is mostly used in Chinese cooking and also in many Indonesian countries and Goa. It has a flavour similar to aniseed but much stronger. The commonest use is in Chinese five-spice powder and is often added to dishes of roast meat and poultry.

JUNIPER BERRIES

Although dried juniper berries are added to many dishes, probably the commonest use is in making gin! They are used in Central Europe in terrines and marinades, and are particularly common with game and pork dishes. Although in Britain they are used mainly for spicing beef, they are a particularly common ingredient with game dishes to complement the strong flavour of the meat.

NUTMEG

Although nutmeg is used commonly in sweet dishes such as rice pudding, it also adds a wonderful flavour to vegetables such as spinach, cauliflower, potato and onion, and can be added to milk sauces. The nutmeg is best bought whole and finely grated fresh, as ground nutmeg tends to lose its flavour very quickly.

ALLSPICE

Allspice is usually used in sweet dishes such as cakes and puddings, whereas in the Middle East it is used in savoury dishes such as game and mince. It is a very good additive for pâtés.

PEPPER

Pepper is without question the best known of all the spices. Both black and white peppercorns should be freshly ground for maximal effect, as the ground variety soon loses its quality. It has the advantage of spicing up any dish. The only advantage of white peppercorns over black is their aesthetic appearance, although black peppercorns have a much stronger flavour.

SESAME SEEDS

Sesame seeds are most commonly ground into oils: a light refined oil for salad dressing, and a rich olive oil (which is much more dense in flavour) made from the toasted seeds. Sesame is most commonly known for its association with tahini, the base of many spreads such as hummus (made with chickpeas), and also toasted sesame seeds are commonly scattered over salads or in Chinese dishes.

MUSTARD SEEDS

There are several different types of mustard seeds, and this accounts for the different flavours of mustard. The commonest use is as a paste to spice up any dish, particularly roast beef. For those not requiring such a hot stimulant, German mustard is probably a good alternative as it is made with white mustard seeds only, with some sugar and herbs. In many Indian dishes, ground mustard seeds are cooked with fish and vegetable dishes and prepared mustard is commonly utilised in many French dishes such as casseroles and sauces.

WASABI

Although commonly thought of as a Japanese horseradish, in fact wasabi is not a true horseradish plant. It is actually more associated botanically with watercress. Its most common use is as an accompaniment to sushi and sashimi and it is also used as a dipping sauce with mirin and soy sauce.

GINGER

One of the great giants of the spices, ginger has more uses than can easily be enumerated. Although commonly available as a ground spice, it is by far the healthiest and tastiest when freshly added to many dishes. It is somewhere between a herb and a spice. Although commonest in dishes from the Middle East and the Far East, it is particularly used in the UK to spice wine.

Spice mixtures

Although to the true gourmet spice mixtures are not acceptable, for those of us in the real world they can add tremendous speed and value to the production of wonderful meals.

GARAM MASALA

Garam masala is probably the commonest spice mixture from Northern India. It includes ground coriander seeds, cumin seeds, cinnamon, cloves, peppercorns, cardamom, nutmeg and bay leaves.

HARISSA

Harissa is commonly served with couscous in Morocco. It includes chilli peppers, salt, garlic, caraway seeds and obviously olive oil.

CURRY POWDER

Curry powder is a European development in Indian curries to avoid the tedious process of grinding all the ingredients together. It includes cumin seeds, coriander seeds, black peppercorns, black mustard seeds, cardamom, fenugreek, turmeric, ginger and chilli powder. It can easily be seen why many people prefer the quicker option of curry powder rather than the more tedious manufacture of individually ground ingredients – although the latter are infinitely better!

CHINESE FIVE SPICE

Chinese five spice is probably characterised mostly by star anise, which has a very strong liquorice flavour. It also includes cloves, Szechuan pepper, fennel and cinnamon. Its strong flavour is a common accompaniment to many Chinese dishes.

Chart your progress!

Before commencing the programme, the first step towards changing your nutritional habits would be to take a very simple nutritional questionnaire.

Cooking is boring
    Yes   No

Cooking is too time-consuming
    Yes   No

Food is too expensive
    Yes   No

No time for this
    Yes   No

Time constraints
    Yes   No

Things that could prevent you changing your nutritional choices:

Are you at the top of your career ladder?
   Yes   No

In transition (a more sedentary way of life)?
   Yes   No

Settled in a job (which means stuck in the old routine)?
   Yes   No

Empty nest (children left home, new organisational skills required)?
   Yes   No

Score 1 point for every Yes and 0 for every No in the above questionnaire. If you have scored more than 3, you have a problem!

Fortunately the recipes that follow are the ideal solution to resolving the problem! The recipes have been deliberately selected for their nutritional content and – most importantly – for their taste! However, the *timing* of the meals is not intended to be carved in stone: for example, suggestions for breakfast (such as poached eggs or toasted cheese) are equally suitable as a light supper. How you adapt these suggestions to your own lifestyle is entirely personal preference.

We have deliberately emphasised certain foods more than others: there are more recipes for fish and poultry than for red meat. Salad ideas are plentiful. This is a positive bias not a negative bias: as you age, deficiencies of certain vitamins and minerals become more common, so it is important to positively emphasise the importance of fatty fish (for vitamin D, deficiency leading to osteoporosis) and eggs (a high source of vitamin B12) to help prevent medical conditions commonly associated with the ageing process.

BREAKFAST

Scottish porridge

For 2

100 g organic oatmeal

150 ml milk

500 ml boiling water

tsp salt

Mix together the oatmeal and milk in a medium mixing bowl to form a paste, then stir in the boiling water.

Transfer to medium saucepan and simmer for 15 minutes, occasionally stirring.

Sprinkle over salt, and serve.

Carbohydrate content per serving: 38 g

Poached eggs

For 2

2 large free-range eggs
2 slices of buttered wholemeal toast

Fill a medium saucepan with water and bring to the boil, then reduce to a simmer.

Break each egg separately into a cup and slide the eggs into the boiling water.

Cook for approximately 3 minutes, then remove the eggs with a slotted spoon.

Serve each egg on a slice of buttered wholemeal toast.

Carbohydrate content per serving: 17 g

Toasted cheese

For 2

2 slices of buttered wholemeal toast
2 tbsp freshly grated cheese (Gouda, Emmental,
Jarlsberg or Cheddar)
freshly ground black pepper

Toast the wholemeal bread then butter lightly.

Spread the grated cheese over the toast and return to the grill until the cheese has melted.

This meal can be augmented quite simply by many different additions, such as:

1 tbsp herbs such as basil, coriander or chives
cherry tomatoes, diced
sliced prosciutto ham
1 tsp Worcestershire sauce
dill and smoked salmon

Carbohydrate content per serving: 16 g

Omelette

For 2

4 large free-range eggs
1 tbsp full cream milk
freshly ground black pepper
25 g unsalted butter

Beat the eggs in a mixing bowl with the milk and season to taste.

Heat the butter in an omelette pan, add the egg mixture and cook on high for about a minute, then gently lift the edge of the omelette to allow the egg to cook more rapidly.

As the egg begins to set, fold the side of the omelette to the centre and serve.

Of course that was a plain omelette, however there are many other potential ways to improve this by adding:

smoked salmon with dill
freshly grated cheese, such as Cheddar, Gruyère or Jarlsberg
chopped fresh herbs such as basil
cherry tomatoes and chives
Parma ham

Carbohydrate content per serving: 3 g

Breakfast platter

For 2

A selection of cold meats, with eggs, nuts and fruit

Almost all the ingredients are ready to eat, with very little prepa-ration, and therefore this is the ultimate fast-food breakfast. A simple selection may include:

one piece of fruit (avoiding mangos, banana and pineapple)
cooked meats such as turkey, chicken, ham or beef
pre-cooked fish, such as smoked trout or mackerel
smoked salmon
cooked chicken
nuts (avoiding cashews, macadamia and chestnuts)
hard-boiled eggs
natural cheeses

Carbohydrate content per serving: nil (excluding fruit)

Fresh fruit with natural yoghurt

For 2

50 g fresh strawberries
50 g fresh blueberries
1 medium orange, peeled and chopped
1 medium peach, stone removed and flesh chopped
100 ml natural yoghurt

Mix together the fruit and berries in a medium bowl.

Transfer to small bowls and pour over the yoghurt.

Carbohydrate content per serving: 22 g

Avocado and toast

For 2

1 medium, ripe Hass avocado, peeled, stone removed
and flesh sliced
2 slices of toasted wholemeal bread
1 tsp Tabasco sauce
freshly ground black pepper

Spread the avocado slices over the toast liberally.

Drizzle over the Tabasco sauce, season to taste.

Carbohydrate content per serving: 18 g

Scrambled eggs with basil and oregano

For 2

50 g unsalted butter

2 medium organic tomatoes, chopped

1 small garlic clove, peeled and chopped finely

2 tsp chopped fresh basil leaves

2 tsp chopped fresh oregano

4 large free-range eggs, beaten

pinch of sea salt

freshly ground black pepper

Melt the butter in a medium frying pan, then gently sauté the tomatoes and garlic for 2–3 minutes.

Add the basil, oregano and eggs, season to taste, and cook over medium heat.

When almost set, but still creamy, serve.

Carbohydrate content per serving: 4 g

Berry smoothie

For 2

100 g blueberries

100 g raspberries

1 tbsp freshly squeezed lemon juice

100 ml mineral water

Blend together the blueberries, raspberries and lemon juice. Dilute to taste and serve.

Carbohydrate content per serving: 10 g

Strawberry and orange smoothie

For 2

100 g strawberries
100 ml natural yoghurt
100 ml freshly squeezed orange juice

Blend together strawberries and yoghurt.

Blend in the orange juice and serve.

Carbohydrate content per serving: 9 g

SOUPS

Pumpkin and ginger soup

For 2

2 tbsp extra-virgin olive oil

1 medium white onion, peeled and diced

750 g butternut pumpkin, peeled and chopped

1 tsp ground cumin

½ tsp ground turmeric

400 ml vegetable bouillon

1 tbsp chopped fresh coriander

2 slices of fresh ginger root, peeled and chopped finely

pinch of sea salt

freshly ground black pepper

100 ml cream

1 tbsp chopped fresh chives

Heat the extra-virgin olive oil in a large saucepan and sauté the onion and pumpkin for 3 minutes.

Stir in the cumin and turmeric, and sauté for a further 2 minutes.

Add the bouillon, coriander and ginger, bring to the boil, and simmer for 20 minutes.

Transfer to a blender and purée, then return to the saucepan.

Season to taste, stir in about 80 ml of cream, and heat through gently.

Serve immediately with a swirl of cream, and garnish with freshly chopped chives.

Carbohydrate content per serving: 15 g

Broccoli and lemon mint soup

For 2

25 g unsalted butter

1 medium red onion, peeled and diced

1 garlic clove, peeled and chopped finely

400 ml vegetable bouillon

250 g broccoli florets

2 tbsp chopped fresh lemon mint leaves

pinch of sea salt

freshly ground black pepper

1 tbsp freshly grated Parmesan cheese

Melt the butter in a large saucepan and sauté the onion and garlic for 2–3 minutes.

Add the vegetable bouillon and slowly bring to the boil.

Stir in the broccoli florets and mint, season to taste, and gently simmer for 15–20 minutes.

Remove from the heat and allow to cool.

Blend to a smooth purée and check the seasoning.

Heat through before serving, garnished with grated Parmesan.

Carbohydrate content per serving: 3 g

Courgette and basil soup

For 2

1 tbsp olive oil

3 medium courgettes, chopped

1 garlic clove, peeled and chopped finely

300 ml vegetable stock

2 tsp Parmesan cheese, grated

handful of basil leaves

1 tbsp crème fraîche

Add the olive oil to a medium saucepan, heat the oil then add the courgettes and garlic.

Sauté the courgettes in garlic for about 10–15 minutes.

Add the stock and bring to the boil, then reduce to simmer for about 5 minutes.

Season to taste with sea salt and freshly ground black pepper.

Stir in the Parmesan, basil and crème fraîche.

Transfer the mixture to a blender and blend.

Serve, garnished with some grated Parmesan cheese.

Carbohydrate content per serving: 5 g

Mussel soup with lime and coriander

For 4

1 kg fresh mussels

800 ml chicken stock

1 red chilli, deseeded and chopped

juice of 2 limes

handful of fresh coriander leaves

sea salt

freshly ground black pepper

Scrub the mussels to remove the fibrous beards.

Discard any mussels that are broken or open.

If any mussels are open, tap them gently to check that they are able to close, otherwise discard.

Place mussels in a large saucepan and add hot water then boil for 4–5 minutes.

Drain the mussels and remove from their shells, then set aside.

In a separate pan, bring the stock to the boil, then add chilli, lime juice and coriander.

Add the mussels, and simmer for 2 minutes.

Season to taste.

Carbohydrate content per serving: 6 g

White onion soup with goat's cheese

For 2

25 g unsalted butter

300 g white onion, peeled and sliced

sprig of thyme

50 ml dry white wine

250 ml chicken stock

100 ml crème fraîche

50 g mature goat's cheese, preferably as a log, sliced into rounds

Tabasco sauce

chives, snipped

Melt butter in a medium saucepan then gently sauté the onions and thyme.

Sweat for about 10 minutes, stirring frequently.

Add the wine, turn the heat up to simmer and reduce by about half.

Stir in the chicken stock, and simmer for about 10 minutes.

Discard the thyme and purée with the crème fraîche.

Season to taste.

Add a swirl of crème fraîche, top with goat's cheese rounds, add a dash of Tabasco and sprinkle over the chives.

Carbohydrate content per serving: 10 g

FISH AND SHELLFISH

Smoked salmon frittata

For 2

4 large free-range eggs, beaten

100 g smoked salmon, finely sliced

1 tbsp chopped fresh dill

1 tbsp chopped fresh chives

pinch of sea salt

freshly ground black pepper

2 tbsp extra-virgin olive oil

sprigs of fresh dill, to garnish

100 g spinach leaves, washed

Mix together the eggs, smoked salmon, dill and chives, and season to taste.

Heat the extra-virgin olive oil in a medium frying pan and pour in the egg mixture.

Cook over low heat for about 5–6 minutes.

When almost set, place under a grill for 2 minutes.

Garnish with sprigs of fresh dill and serve on a bed of spinach leaves.

Carbohydrate content per serving: negligible

Oat-crusted cod

For 2

½ tbsp flour

1 tbsp oatmeal

1 tbsp porridge oats

1 tbsp chopped fresh basil leaves

Sea salt

Freshly ground black pepper

2 cod fillets, approx 150 g each

50 ml full cream milk

extra-virgin olive oil

Mix together the flour, oatmeal, porridge, basil and seasoning in a medium bowl.

Coat the fish with the milk, then coat with the oatmeal mixture.

Shallow fry the fish in olive oil for about two minutes per side.

Serve immediately.

Carbohydrate content per serving: 14 g

Smoked trout with watercress and mint sauce

For 2

watercress and mint sauce

2 smoked trout fillets

fresh mint, to garnish

lemon wedges

pinch of sea salt

freshly ground black pepper

Watercress and mint sauce

1 tbsp fresh watercress leaves, chopped

2 tbsp fresh mint leaves, chopped

100 ml natural yoghurt

1 tbsp freshly squeezed lemon juice

pinch of cayenne pepper

Mix together the ingredients for the sauce, and chill in the fridge for 2 hours.

Serve the trout, pour over the watercress and mint sauce, season and garnish with fresh mint leaves and lemon wedges.

Carbohydrate content per serving: 5 g

Salmon steak parcels

For 2

2 salmon steaks, approximately 150–175 g each

2 tbsp extra-virgin olive oil

pinch of rock salt

freshly ground black pepper

1 tbsp chopped fresh dill

1 tbsp chopped fresh chives

1 tbsp freshly squeezed lime juice

lime wedges

stir-fried vegetables with sesame seeds

Place the salmon steaks on individual sheets of aluminium foil, and brush with extra-virgin olive oil.

Season to taste and sprinkle the dill and chives over the salmon.

Close the foil parcels and cook in the centre of a pre-heated oven at 180°C (gas mark 4) for about 20 minutes.

Remove the salmon from the parcels and drizzle over freshly squeezed lime juice.

Serve immediately with lime wedges and stir-fried vegetables with sesame seeds.

Carbohydrate content per serving: 26 g

(1 g without vegetables)

Spicy whiting with courgette and parsley salad

For 2

1 tsp ground cumin seeds

1 tsp ground coriander seeds

1 tsp turmeric

2 large free-range eggs, beaten

1 small white onion, peeled and grated

1 garlic clove, peeled and grated

2 slices of fresh ginger root, peeled and grated

2 tsp freshly squeezed lemon juice

pinch of sea salt

freshly ground black pepper

4 medium whiting fillets, approximately 75 g each

2 tbsp plain flour

4 tbsp extra-virgin olive oil

fresh coriander leaves

courgette and parsley salad (page 225)

Dry stir-fry the ground cumin, coriander and turmeric in a small frying pan over medium heat for about a minute, then set aside to cool.

Mix together the beaten eggs with the onion, garlic, ginger, cumin, coriander, turmeric and lemon juice, and season to taste.

Coat the fillets with the egg mixture, then dust with flour.

Heat the extra-virgin olive oil in a medium frying pan and fry the fish for about 2 minutes per side, turning once.

Garnish with fresh coriander leaves, and serve with courgette and parsley salad.

Carbohydrate content per serving: 15 g
(including salad)

Tuna steaks with asparagus

For 2

2 tbsp extra-virgin olive oil

2 medium tuna steaks, approximately 150 g each

small bunch of asparagus, washed and trimmed

lemon wedges

pinch of rock salt

freshly ground black pepper

Heat the olive oil in a medium saucepan then sear the tuna over a high heat for about 4 minutes, turning once.

Remove from high heat, and fry over a medium heat for about 4 minutes, turning once, or slightly longer depending on personal taste.

At the same time

Lightly steam the asparagus.

Serve the tuna with lightly steamed asparagus and lemon wedges, and season to taste.

Carbohydrate content per serving: 4 g

Calamari and ginger

For 2

2 tbsp extra-virgin olive oil

1 tsp toasted sesame oil

75 g spring onions, chopped (on the diagonal) into 3–4 cm lengths

3 slices of fresh ginger root, peeled and chopped finely

1 sweet red pepper, deseeded and chopped

150 g fresh calamari tubes, sliced into rings

1 tbsp light soy sauce

juice of a freshly squeezed orange

freshly ground black pepper

1 pak choi, halved

Heat the extra-virgin olive oil and sesame oil in a wok, and sauté the spring onions for about a minute.

Add the ginger, pepper and calamari, and stir-fry for 3–4 minutes.

Stir in the soy sauce and orange juice, season to taste, and cook for a final 1–2 minutes.

At the same time

Lightly steam the pak choi.

Serve the calamari on the pak choi.

Carbohydrate content per serving: 6 g

Chilli prawns with pepper

For 2

2 tbsp extra-virgin olive oil

1 shallot, peeled and diced

1 garlic clove, peeled and chopped

1 small red chilli, deseeded and chopped

1 medium yellow pepper, deseeded and finely sliced

250 g cooked tiger prawns, shelled

1 tbsp soy sauce

1 tbsp fresh coriander leaves, chopped

freshly ground black pepper

Heat the olive oil in a medium frying pan and sauté the shallot, garlic, chilli and pepper for 2 minutes.

Add the prawns, soy sauce and coriander and season to taste.

Stir-fry for a further 2 minutes and serve immediately.

Carbohydrate content per serving: 4 g

MEAT

Halloumi and tomato kebabs

For 2

125 g halloumi cheese, cubed

8 organic cherry tomatoes

4 rashers of pancetta

1 tbsp chopped fresh coriander

fresh coriander, to garnish

Soak 4 wooden skewers for 2 hours before use (preferably overnight).

Divide the cheese into small cubes. Halloumi is a firm cheese, so this is relatively easy.

Thread the cubes of cheese and cherry tomatoes alternately on the skewers, and grill under a medium grill (8–10 cm from the grill) for 4–5 minutes, turning once.

At the same time

Lightly grill the pancetta for 3–4 minutes, turning once.

Top with chopped fresh coriander and serve the kebabs and pancetta immediately, garnished with sprigs of fresh coriander.

Carbohydrate content per serving: 5 g

Lamb cutlets with garlic butter sauce

For 2

6 medium lean lamb cutlets

2 tbsp extra-virgin olive oil

75 g broccoli florets

75 g yellow squash

75 g unsalted butter

2 garlic cloves, peeled and finely chopped

freshly ground black pepper

sprigs of fresh mint, to garnish

Brush the cutlets on both sides with extra-virgin olive oil, and cook under a hot grill, for 4–5 minutes, turning once.

Lightly steam the broccoli and squash.

Heat the butter in a small saucepan, sauté the garlic until softened, and season to taste.

Serve the cutlets with the garlic butter sauce and vegetables, garnished with fresh mint.

Carbohydrate content per serving: 7 g

Steak with salsa verde

For 2

1 tbsp fresh flat-leaf parsley, chopped

1 tbsp fresh basil leaves, chopped

1 tbsp fresh oregano leaves, chopped

1 clove garlic, peeled and chopped finely

1 anchovy fillet, rinsed and chopped

1 dsp red wine vinegar

1 dsp freshly squeezed lemon juice

1 dsp wholegrain mustard

2 tbsp extra-virgin olive oil

pinch of sea salt

freshly ground black pepper

2 fillet steaks (150 g)

In a small mixing bowl, mix together the parsley, basil, oregano, garlic and anchovy.

Add the red wine vinegar, lemon juice, mustard and one tablespoon olive oil.

Season to taste with salt and pepper and set aside.

Add the remaining olive oil to a medium frying pan and fry the fillet steaks for 1–2 minutes each side.

Spoon over the salsa verde.

Carbohydrate content per serving: 3 g

Slow-cooked lamb and rosemary

For 4

2 tbsp extra-virgin olive oil

1.5 kg lamb (for oven-cooking), cubed

2 tbsp plain flour

3 tbsp freshly chopped rosemary

3 red onions, sliced

2 garlic cloves, peeled and chopped finely

1 small aubergine, cubed

2 medium courgettes, chopped on the diagonal

2 tbsp tomato purée

300 ml vegetable bouillon

pinch of sea salt

freshly ground black pepper

Heat the extra-virgin olive oil in a large pan over a medium heat.

At the same time, place the lamb cubes into a large mixing bowl, and toss with flour, rosemary and seasoning.

Fry the lamb for about 5 minutes in the oil until brown.

Remove from the pan and set aside.

Add the onions, garlic, aubergine and courgettes to the pan.

Fry for about 5–6 minutes until golden brown.

Return the lamb to the pan with the tomato purée and stir in the stock.

Cover the pot and simmer for about one hour until the lamb is tender.

Season to taste.

Carbohydrate content per serving: 15 g

Spicy beef patties

For 2

1 small red onion, peeled and diced

1 garlic clove, peeled and chopped finely

1 red chilli, deseeded and chopped

1 stick lemongrass, peeled and chopped finely

2 tbsp fresh coriander leaves, chopped finely

2 slices fresh ginger root, peeled and chopped finely

250 g steak mince

1 egg yolk

pinch of sea salt

freshly ground black pepper

2 tbsp extra-virgin olive oil

handful of peppery watercress, washed

20 g sesame seeds, toasted

Mix together the onion, garlic, chilli, lemongrass, coriander and ginger in a large mixing bowl.

Stir in the steak mince and egg yolk then season to taste.

Shape into patties.

Heat the extra-virgin olive oil in a large frying pan and fry the patties for about 3 minutes each side.

Serve on a bed of peppery watercress and sprinkle over toasted sesame seeds.

Carbohydrate content per serving: 3 g

Cubetti di pancetta tomatoes

For 2

1 garlic clove, peeled and chopped finely

1 tbsp of chopped fresh basil

1 tbsp of chopped fresh flat-leaf parsley

2 beefsteak tomatoes, halved

1 tbsp of cubetti di pancetta

1 tbsp extra-virgin olive oil

1 tbsp Parmesan flakes

pinch of sea salt

freshly ground black pepper

Mix together the garlic, basil and parsley.

Add 3–4 tablespoons of water to a shallow casserole dish then place the tomatoes (cut side uppermost) in the dish.

Place half the garlic and herb mixture on each tomato, top with cubetti di pancetta and drizzle a little extra-virgin olive oil on the tomatoes and top with Parmesan flakes.

Bake in the centre of a pre-heated oven at 180°C (gas mark 4) for 10–12 minutes and season.

Carbohydrate content per serving: 6 g

POULTRY

Chicken paprika

For 2

2 chicken breasts, about 150 g each

50 g butter, cubed

2 tbsp extra-virgin olive oil

1 medium brown onion, peeled and sliced

1 garlic clove, peeled and chopped finely

1 tbsp plain flour

1 tbsp paprika

100 ml chicken stock

1 beefsteak tomato, peeled and chopped

2 tsp tomato purée

freshly ground black pepper

100 g open-cup mushrooms, wiped and halved lengthways

75 g French beans

150 ml natural yoghurt

sprigs of fresh tarragon, to garnish

Place the chicken fillets in a shallow baking dish, dot with butter cubes, and bake in the centre of a pre-heated oven at 180°C (gas mark 4) for 20–25 minutes.

Remove from the oven and allow to cool, then slice into thin strips.

Heat the extra-virgin olive oil in a medium frying pan and sauté the onion and garlic for 1–2 minutes.

Add the chicken to the pan, and stir in the flour and paprika.

Stir in the stock, tomato and tomato purée, season to taste, and simmer for 10 minutes.

Add the mushrooms and simmer for a further 5 minutes.

At the same time

Lightly steam the French beans.

Stir in the natural yoghurt to the chicken paprika in the pan, and heat through gently.

Serve with French beans, garnished with sprigs of fresh tarragon.

Carbohydrate content per serving: 20 g

Tarragon chicken

For 4

100 g unsalted butter

2 tbsp freshly squeezed lemon juice

2 garlic cloves, peeled and finely chopped

2 tbsp fresh tarragon, chopped

4 tbsp flat-leaf parsley, chopped

pinch of sea salt

freshly ground black pepper

1.5 kg chicken

Mix together the butter, lemon juice, garlic, herbs and seasoning in a bowl.

Loosen the chicken skin gently over the legs and breast and smooth the herb butter under the skin.

Season skin with sea salt and freshly ground black pepper.

Place the chicken on a roasting tray in the centre of a pre-heated oven at 200°C (gas mark 6) and roast for 30 minutes.

Baste the chicken with the juices then roast for another 30 minutes.

Remove from the oven and allow to settle for 15 minutes before serving.

Carbohydrate content per serving: 1 g

Duck with mango purée

For 2

2 Gressingham duck breast fillets
1 medium ripe mango
3 tbsp freshly squeezed lime juice
3 slices fresh ginger root, peeled and chopped finely
1 green chilli, deseeded and chopped finely
1 tbsp chopped fresh coriander leaves
pinch of sea salt
freshly ground black pepper
sprigs of redcurrants

Pre-heat oven to 200°C (gas mark 6).

Place the duck breasts on a roasting tin, skin side down, slashing the skin beforehand.

Cook in the centre of the oven for 30 minutes, then remove from the oven and set aside.

Sauce

Peel the mango and purée in a blender with the lime juice and ginger.

Heat the mango purée in a small saucepan, stirring in the chilli and coriander.

Slice the duck breasts and drizzle over the mango purée.

Serve with sprigs of redcurrants.

Carbohydrate content per serving: 14 g

Guinea fowl with leeks

For 2

1 guinea fowl

2 level tbsp seasoned plain flour

2 tbsp extra-virgin olive oil

4 shallots, peeled and chopped

1 garlic clove, peeled and crushed

2 leeks, trimmed and sliced finely

100 ml white wine, preferably dry

200 ml vegetable bouillon

50 ml single cream

1 tbsp chopped fresh basil leaves

pinch of sea salt

freshly ground black pepper

Pre-heat oven to 180°C (gas mark 4).

Remove the drumsticks and thighs and breasts from the guinea fowl.

Toss the drumsticks, thighs and breasts in the seasoned flour.

Heat 1 tablespoon of extra-virgin olive oil in a large frying pan and lightly sauté the guinea fowl until browned.

Transfer to a large casserole dish.

Heat the remaining tablespoon of oil in the pan on a moderate heat and sauté the shallots and garlic for 2–3 minutes.

Transfer to the casserole with the guinea fowl.

Place the leeks in the frying pan and sauté gently for about 4–5 minutes, then transfer to the casserole.

Stir the wine and bouillon into the casserole and place in the oven for about an hour, stirring occasionally.

Remove the guinea fowl from the casserole and reduce the liquid over a high heat for about 10 minutes then stir in the cream.

Stir in the basil, season to taste and serve over the guinea fowl.

Carbohydrate content per serving: 24 g

Poached chicken with spring vegetables

For 4

1 free-range chicken, approx 1.5 kg, skin on

25 g fresh sage

25 g fresh flat-leaf parsley, chopped

pinch of sea salt

freshly ground black pepper

2 tbsp extra-virgin olive oil

8 small organic carrots, scraped, and topped and tailed

2 yellow squash, halved

4 asparagus tips

2 leeks, washed, trimmed and chopped

1 tbsp lemon juice

Score the chicken breast and place the sage and parsley under the skin.

Season the chicken.

Brush the skin with the extra-virgin olive oil.

Place the chicken on a roasting tray in the centre of a pre-heated oven at 200°C (gas mark 6) and roast for 30 minutes.

Baste the chicken with the juices then roast for another 30 minutes.

Remove from the oven and allow to rest for 15 minutes before serving.

At the same time (about 15 minutes before chicken is ready)

Lightly steam the vegetables and drizzle over the lemon juice.

Carbohydrate content per serving: 14 g

Chicken with rosemary and thyme

For 2

1 garlic clove, peeled and chopped finely

sea salt

2 medium chicken breasts

1 tbsp extra-virgin olive oil

2 sprigs rosemary

2 sprigs thyme

freshly ground black pepper

2 tbsp almond flakes

Pre-heat oven to 200°C (gas mark 6).

Rub the garlic and salt into the chicken breasts.

Place the chicken in a shallow baking dish and drizzle with oil.

Add rosemary and thyme.

Bake in the pre-heated oven for about 20 minutes, basting occasionally.

Sprinkle over the almond flakes.

Season to taste and serve immediately.

Carbohydrate content per serving: 2 g

Pheasant with lemon butter and French beans

For 2

2 tbsp extra-virgin olive oil

1 pheasant

6 pancetta slices

2 shallots, peeled and sliced

2 garlic cloves, peeled and chopped

2 tbsp sage leaves, chopped finely

200 ml Sauvignon blanc

50 g unsalted butter

2 tbsp freshly squeezed lemon juice

100 g French beans

pinch of sea salt

freshly ground black pepper

Pre-heat oven to 180°C (gas mark 4).

In a casserole dish heat the olive oil and brown the pheasant.

Wrap the pancetta around the pheasant then add the shallots, garlic and sage.

Add the wine, cover and cook in the pre-heated oven for 30 minutes, basting occasionally.

Melt the butter in a medium saucepan, add the lemon juice and beans and cook for 2–3 minutes.

Serve the pheasant with the French beans and season to taste.

Carbohydrate content per serving: 8 g

SALADS

Asparagus and rocket salad

For 2

4 asparagus spears

1 cup of fresh peas

1 cup of broad beans

large handful of wild rocket

1 tbsp extra-virgin olive oil

small bunch of flat-leaf parsley leaves

1 tbsp Pecorino cheese, flaked

drizzle of balsamic vinegar

Top and tail the asparagus and slice on the diagonal.

Blanche the asparagus in hot water for about 2 minutes, then set aside to drain.

Blanche the fresh peas for about 2 minutes.

Blanche the broad beans.

Mix together the rocket, asparagus, beans and peas, then dress with some seasoning and the extra-virgin olive oil.

Arrange the mixture on the plate, then garnish with parsley, Pecorino and a drizzle of balsamic vinegar.

Carbohydrate content per serving: 7 g

Courgette and lemon salad

For 2

2 medium courgettes, shaved lengthways

zest of 1 lemon

zest of 1 lime

2 tsp lemon juice

2 tsp lime juice

1 tbsp extra-virgin olive oil

1 tbsp tarragon

1 tsp runny honey

small handful pine nuts

Mix together the courgettes, zest of lemon and lime in a bowl.

In a separate bowl, mix together the lemon and lime juice, olive oil, tarragon and honey.

Season to taste.

Drizzle the dressing over the courgettes.

Sprinkle over the pine nuts.

Carbohydrate content per serving: 9 g

Stilton and toasted walnut pâté

For 4

100 g Stilton cheese, crumbled

50 g Camembert

1 tsp port

½ tsp ground nutmeg

50 g walnuts, toasted and chopped

Mix together the cheese, port, nutmeg and walnuts.

Transfer to a sheet of greaseproof paper and arrange into a rectangle.

Transfer to the fridge for 2 hours to chill.

Carbohydrate content per serving: 2 g

Blueberry and mint salad

For 2

1 medium red onion, peeled and sliced into rings

1½ tbsp extra-virgin olive oil

75 g baby spinach leaves

100 g fresh blueberries, washed

125 g goat's cheese (or Wigmore ewe's milk cheese)

handful of fresh mint leaves

1 tbsp white wine vinegar

sea salt

freshly ground black pepper

Pre-heat oven to 180°C (gas mark 4).

Place the onion rings in an ovenproof dish, drizzle with 1 tablespoon of olive oil and sear in the oven for 6–8 minutes.

Mix together the spinach leaves, blueberries, cheese and mint in a salad bowl.

Separately mix together the white wine vinegar, a teaspoon of olive oil, and season.

Place the onion in the centre of the plate and top with the blueberry and mint salad.

Serve immediately.

Carbohydrate content per serving: 6 g

Halloumi and fennel salad

For 2

1 fennel bulb

50 g crème fraîche

1 garlic clove, crushed

2 tsp extra-virgin olive oil

100 g wild rocket leaves, washed

juice of 1 lemon

100 g halloumi, cubed

seeds of 1 pomegranate

Slice the fennel thinly.

Whisk the crème fraîche with the garlic and a teaspoon of olive oil, season to taste and set aside.

Toss the rocket with the lemon juice in a salad bowl.

Add a teaspoon of extra-virgin olive oil to a medium frying pan and cook the halloumi for 2–3 minutes.

Sprinkle the halloumi over the salad and sprinkle over the pomegranate seeds.

Drizzle over the cream dressing.

Carbohydrate content per serving: 8 g

Aubergines with yoghurt and cucumber

For 2

4 aubergines

1 tbsp extra-virgin olive oil

1 small cucumber, grated

100 g natural yoghurt

garlic clove, peeled and crushed

small handful of mint leaves, washed

Pre-heat oven to 180°C (gas mark 4).

Halve the aubergines lengthways.

Place the aubergines in a baking tray and drizzle over a tablespoon of extra-virgin olive oil.

Place in the oven and cook for about 30–40 minutes.

Cucumber and yoghurt

Place the cucumber in a bowl.

Stir in the yoghurt, garlic and mint leaves.

Serve the aubergines topped with cucumber mint yoghurt.

Carbohydrate content per serving: 20 g

Rocket and olive salad

For 2

100 g wild rocket leaves, washed

2 tsp capers, rinsed

50 g green olives

2 anchovy fillets, chopped

1 tbsp chopped fresh mint leaves

freshly ground black pepper

60 ml garlic vinaigrette

Mix together the rocket, capers, olives, anchovies and mint, and season to taste.

Drizzle over the garlic vinaigrette.

Carbohydrate content per serving: 1 g

Chicken and pine nut salad

For 2

2 organic chicken breast fillets, approximately 125 g each

200 g spinach leaves, washed

1 Lebanese cucumber, sliced lengthways

2 spring onions, chopped on the diagonal

1 tbsp chopped fresh basil

50 g raw pine nuts

freshly ground black pepper

Lemon and coriander vinaigrette

3 tbsp extra-virgin olive oil

1 tsp white wine vinegar

½ garlic clove, peeled and grated

2 tsp lemon juice

2 tsp chopped fresh coriander leaves

freshly ground black pepper

Place the chicken fillets in a shallow oven-safe dish and dot with butter.

Cover with perforated aluminium foil and cook in the centre of a pre-heated oven at 180°C (gas mark 4) for 20–25 minutes.

At the same time

Prepare the vinaigrette.

Mix together the ingredients in a screw-top jar and shake vigorously.

Remove the chicken from the oven, set aside to cool then slice.

Arrange the spinach on the plates. Toss the cucumber, spring onions and basil with the pine nuts, then season and serve on the bed of spinach.

Top with chicken and drizzle over the dressing.

Carbohydrate content per serving: 6 g

Chicken, artichoke and pancetta salad

For 2

2 medium organic chicken breasts

2 Jerusalem artichokes, peeled

1 tbsp butter

1 tbsp extra-virgin olive oil

1 tbsp sage leaves, chopped

100 g cubetti di pancetta

handful of wild rocket leaves

pinch of sea salt

freshly ground black pepper

Passata vinaigrette

For 2

3 tbsp extra-virgin olive oil

3 tbsp passata

1 tbsp red wine vinegar

small garlic clove, peeled and grated

pinch of sea salt

freshly ground black pepper

Pre-heat oven to 200°C (gas mark 6) and cook the chicken breasts for about 20 minutes.

Remove from the oven and set aside.

Slice the artichokes thinly and blanch in salty boiling water.

Remove and drain.

At the same time

Prepare the vinaigrette.

Add the ingredients of the vinaigrette to a screw-top jar and shake vigorously.

Add the butter and olive oil to a large non-stick frying pan.

Add the artichoke discs and sage leaves, and sauté for 2–3 minutes.

Set aside and drain.

Slice the chicken breasts.

Mix together the chicken, artichokes, pancetta and sage in a bowl and spoon it over the bed of wild rocket leaves.

Drizzle over the vinaigrette and season to taste.

Carbohydrate content per serving: 10 g

Spinach, orange and fennel salad

For 2

200 g spinach leaves

1 large orange, peeled and segmented

1 fennel bulb, sliced finely

10 g Parmesan cheese, grated finely

Vinaigrette

1 tbsp red wine vinegar

1 tsp sugar

1 tsp Dijon mustard

2 tbsp fresh orange juice

3 tbsp extra-virgin olive oil

sea salt

freshly ground black pepper

Add the red wine vinegar, sugar, mustard, orange juice and oil to a screw-top jar and shake vigorously.

Season to taste with sea salt and freshly ground black pepper and set aside.

In a large mixing bowl, add the spinach leaves, orange and fennel.

Arrange the salad in the centre of the plates, drizzle over the dressing and sprinkle over Parmesan cheese and serve immediately.

It is essential to serve immediately otherwise the fennel will discolour.

Carbohydrate content per serving: 11 g

Avocado, grapefruit and tofu salad

For 2

½ pink grapefruit

2 tbsp extra-virgin olive oil

1 tsp runny honey

½ red chilli, deseeded and finely chopped

2 spring onions, trimmed and sliced on diagonal

50 g tofu, cubed

1 small ripe Hass avocado, peeled and sliced

handful of fresh mint leaves, chopped

lemon and coriander vinaigrette (page 219)

sea salt

freshly ground black pepper

Segment the grapefruit.

Add the grapefruit to the mixing bowl, and stir in the olive oil, honey, chilli and spring onion.

Add the tofu and avocado with the mint leaves.

Toss with the dressing and season to taste.

Carbohydrate content per serving: 10 g

Courgette and parsley salad

For 2

2 medium courgettes

2 yellow summer squash

1 tsp unsalted butter

pinch of sea salt

pinch of coarsely ground black pepper

small handful fresh parsley leaves, chopped

1 tsp grated lemon zest

Slice the courgette and the squash diagonally into 1 cm slices.

In a medium frying pan, melt the butter and add the courgette, squash, salt and pepper.

Cook over a low heat for 5–6 minutes, stirring frequently.

Stir in the parsley and lemon zest and serve immediately.

Carbohydrate content per serving: 5 g

Antipasto salad

For 2

200 g green beans, topped and tailed

1 medium celery stalk, sliced thinly

20 g salami, sliced thinly

100 g mozzarella cheese, sliced

1 medium tomato, sliced

pinch of sea salt

pinch of coarsely ground black pepper

French vinaigrette

For 2

4 tbsp extra-virgin olive oil

1 tbsp white wine vinegar

½ tsp mustard powder

½ garlic clove, peeled and grated

pinch of rock salt

freshly ground black pepper

Prepare the vinaigrette by adding the ingredients to a screw-top jar and shaking vigorously.

Blanch the green beans in boiling water for 2 minutes, then drain. Mix together the green beans, celery, salami, mozzarella and tomato in a large salad bowl, season to taste and drizzle over the vinaigrette.

Carbohydrate content per serving: 6 g

VEGETARIAN

Fennel with Emmental

For 2

2 fennel bulbs

1 tbsp chopped fresh dill

75 g butter, melted

50 g Emmental cheese

freshly ground black pepper

Top and tail the fennel bulbs, cut into segments vertically and lightly steam for 5 minutes.

Place the fennel on a grill tray, sprinkle with fresh chopped dill, then drizzle over the melted butter.

Grate the Emmental over the fennel, then grill until the cheese has melted.

Season with freshly ground black pepper.

Carbohydrate content per serving: 6 g

Leeks in basil mascarpone

For 2

2 leeks, trimmed and sliced lengthways
pinch of sea salt
freshly ground black pepper
1 tbsp chopped fresh basil
100 g mascarpone
pinch of paprika

Lightly steam the leeks until soft, and season.

Stir the fresh basil into the mascarpone.

Spoon the mascarpone over the leeks and dust with paprika.

Carbohydrate content per serving: 4 g

Mushrooms with garlic

For 2

3 tbsp extra-virgin olive oil

1 medium red onion, peeled and sliced

2 garlic cloves, peeled and chopped finely

150 g flat mushrooms, wiped and halved

1 small red chilli, deseeded and chopped

1 tbsp chopped fresh coriander

1 tbsp freshly squeezed lemon juice

freshly ground black pepper

fresh coriander leaves, to garnish

Heat the extra-virgin olive oil in a wok and gently sauté the onion and garlic for 1–2 minutes.

Add the mushrooms, and sauté for a further 3–4 minutes.

Stir in the chilli and coriander, add the lemon juice, and season.

Garnish with fresh coriander leaves.

Carbohydrate content per serving: 5 g

Herb sauce

For 4

1 tbsp freshly chopped flat-leaf parsley
1 tbsp freshly chopped basil
1 tbsp finely chopped fresh oregano
250 g crème fraîche
1 tsp zest of lemon
pinch of rock salt
freshly ground black pepper

Mix together the ingredients in a small mixing bowl.

Herb sauce is particularly suitable for serving with baked chicken or poached salmon.

Carbohydrate content per serving: 6 g

Asparagus with lemon butter sauce

For 2

200 g asparagus, washed and trimmed
75 g butter
2 tbsp freshly squeezed lemon juice
freshly ground black pepper
fresh basil leaves, to garnish

Lightly steam the asparagus.

Melt the butter in a small saucepan, stir in the lemon juice and season to taste.

Arrange the asparagus on warm plates, pour over the lemon butter sauce and garnish with fresh basil.

Carbohydrate content per serving: 4 g

Béarnaise sauce

For 4

3 tbsp tarragon vinegar

half a bay leaf

1 chopped small onion

sprig of chervil

2 fresh organic egg yolks

100 g unsalted butter

sprig of tarragon, leaves chopped

Add the tarragon vinegar, bay leaf, onion and chervil to a small saucepan and bring to the boil.

Reduce by two-thirds and drain before returning to the pan.

Beat two egg yolks and add to the pan whisking over a low heat until thickened.

Add 100 g unsalted butter a little at a time, while whisking continuously.

Increase the heat to thicken the sauce while whisking continuously.

Stir in 1 tablespoon of chopped tarragon and season to taste.

This is particularly suitable over fillets of grilled fish, lamb, or beef.

Carbohydrate content per serving: 4 g

Aubergines with chilli

For 2

1 medium aubergine, chopped into chunks

1 tbsp sea salt

1 tbsp extra-virgin olive oil

2 garlic cloves, peeled and chopped finely

1 small red chilli, deseeded and chopped finely

juice of 1 lemon

handful of parsley leaves, chopped

freshly ground black pepper

Place the aubergine into a colander and sprinkle with the salt and leave for 30 minutes.

Rinse the aubergine thoroughly and pat dry.

Heat the olive oil in a medium frying pan and cook the aubergine for about 3–4 minutes.

Stir in the garlic and chilli and cook for a further 2 minutes.

Stir in the lemon juice and parsley and season to taste.

Serve immediately.

Carbohydrate content per serving: 5 g

Stir-fried vegetables

For 2

1 tbsp sesame seeds

2 tbsp extra-virgin olive oil

1 tsp sesame oil

2 shallots, quartered

2 slices of fresh ginger root, peeled and chopped finely

1 Romano pepper, deseeded and sliced finely

1 small yellow pepper, deseeded and sliced finely

3 medium courgettes, sliced lengthways into matchsticks

3 shiitake mushrooms, wiped and quartered

2 tbsp light soy sauce

2 tbsp mirin (or dry white wine)

freshly ground black pepper

Lightly toast the sesame seeds in a dry pan for about a minute, and set aside.

Heat the extra-virgin olive oil and sesame oil in the wok and sauté the shallots for 1–2 minutes.

Add the ginger, pepper, courgettes and mushrooms.

Stir in the soy sauce and mirin, season to taste, and stir-fry for 3–4 minutes.

Serve with the toasted sesame seeds.

Carbohydrate content per serving: 14 g

Baked tomatoes with basil and garlic

For 2

4 medium-size tomatoes, deseeded

1 tbsp fresh basil leaves, chopped

1 tbsp fresh flat-leaf parsley leaves, chopped

2 garlic cloves, peeled and chopped

20 g fresh breadcrumbs

extra-virgin ollive oil

Place the seeded tomato halves, cut side up, in a medium baking dish.

Mix the herbs and garlic, and spoon into the tomato halves, then top with breadcrumbs.

Drizzle a little extra-virgin olive oil over each tomato half and bake in the oven at about 180°C (gas mark 4) for 1 hour.

Carbohydrate content per serving: 15 g

Sautéed courgettes with garlic and parsley

Persillade is a technique of flavouring sautéed vegetables when they are cooked.

For 2

2 tbsp extra-virgin olive oil

2 large courgettes, topped, tailed and sliced finely

1 garlic clove, grated

1 tbsp fresh flat-leaf parsley, chopped

Heat the extra-virgin olive oil in a moderate saucepan, then lightly fry the courgettes for about 2–3 minutes.

Stir in the garlic and parsley and continue to sauté for another 1–2 minutes.

Serve immediately.

Carbohydrate content per serving: 5 g

Oregano and tomato bagel

For 2

4 medium sun-dried tomatoes, sliced thinly

1 tbsp chopped fresh oregano leaves

freshly ground black pepper

1 medium bagel, halved horizontally

1 tbsp Parmesan flakes

Mix together the sun-dried tomatoes and oregano, and season to taste.

Lightly toast the bagel halves for no more than 1 minute.

Top with the tomato and oregano mixture, sprinkle over the Parmesan flakes, and serve.

Carbohydrate content per serving: 24 g

Eggs Italian-style

For 2

1 tbsp extra-virgin olive oil

1 small red onion, peeled and diced

1 medium garlic clove, peeled and chopped finely

1 beefsteak tomato, chopped

1 tbsp chopped fresh basil

1 tbsp chopped fresh oregano (or ½ tsp dried oregano)

2 large free-range eggs

freshly ground black pepper

Heat the olive oil in a medium frying pan and sauté the onion and garlic for 2–3 minutes.

Stir in the tomato and herbs, and simmer gently for 12–14 minutes.

Crack the eggs separately over the herb tomatoes, in opposite sides of the pan.

Cook for 4–5 minutes.

Season with freshly ground black pepper, and serve immediately.

Carbohydrate content per serving: 5 g

10 Life changes

WITH THE PROGRESS of time, there are many changes that occur in our personal circumstances, from the importance of maintaining mental agility to coping with traumatic events such as grief. The aim of this chapter is to provide practical and effective ways of dealing with the potential changes associated with ageing. Most of the strategies are applicable only in very specific circumstances. Select any – or none – which are appropriate to your personal situation.

The categories which have been examined include:

- Mental agility
- Caring for parents
- Full nest syndrome
- Grandparenting
- Change or departure of parent
- Grief
- New partnership
- Returning to work
- Life outwith the firm

Mental agility

Stopping work brings a loss of mental and social stimulation. It is important to replace this loss, preferably in more enjoyable ways.

Mental workouts

These are not 'brain training' but maintenance of the skills you have.

Mental agility can be exercised alone. Skills are increased by crosswords, word games, Sudoku. Find your daily workout in your newspaper. Look for the right level for you and do not be put off by trying ones that are too difficult. There is a range of computer workouts also.

Bingo helps to maintain the ability to retain numbers, to remain alert and to process new information speedily. Pub quizzes are great at getting the brain working. Scrabble stretches ability with words and has the advantage of sharpening the use of persuasive argument to defend words like *yttria* or *ikat*.

Card-playing has fewer arguments but requires one to think ahead and to second guess the opposition. Dominoes likewise uses the skill of examining possibilities. Theoretically all of these games have a pleasant social side but that depends on how competitive your friends are!

Bridge and chess not only stretch the memory but can be very social. Joining classes or a club is a means of getting to know new people. Bridge is also a game that can be played at different levels. Bridge and chess can be played online at different levels of skill.

Groups: book – and others

The list of special interest groups is endless, their format varied. You name it, you'll find it. The internet or a call to your local radio service are good ways of making contacts. If no book groups exist in your area, try to start one. Check out also organisations such as Probus clubs.

There is always plenty of unpaid work that needs to be done in any community. Look around for something that interests you and decide how much time to give. Groups like Guerrilla Gardening may only operate for a few months. Other activities like canal clearing may be one-offs.

Activities that engage the body as well as the mind give pleasure.

Consider creative classes such as cake decorating, writing, painting and craft. Local Authorities offer an amazing range of interesting classes.

Music-making

Do you know that music-making is one of the best ways to be mentally, physically and socially alive?

Singing has the power to alter mood and has noticeable physical benefits. Find a choir in your neighbourhood. The range of choirs is enormous. Can't play an instrument? Now is the time to learn. It is even possible to learn to play the banjo using the internet.

Dancing is an ideal combination of physical movement, enjoyable social contact plus the pleasurable mental stimulation of learning new dance steps. The complete package.

Caring for parents

Planning ahead for the likelihood of care is the first duty of all family members.

It is a matter of management ability to find a fair, affordable and workable pattern of care. With goodwill, some unselfishness and more imagination solutions can be reached. The earlier such likelihoods are considered the better for all concerned.

ACTION PLAN

1. Explore the availability of government/local provision/social services/respite care/carer support before they are needed. Update this information regularly.
2. Decide how to share the responsibility for delivering this care.
3. Look ahead and agree at what point major changes may have to be made.
4. Identify some likely triggers to future actions.
5. Agree in advance action when the situation is beyond the caring/nursing skills of the family.

Responsibility

Within families sons are notorious for evading the task of caring, claiming job demands, distance, etc., as grounds for undertaking few or no responsibilities. Alternatively they may throw money at the problem.

If geography and employment place burdens on one family member then others have to give up time and money to cover holidays, weekends, financial loss. One daughter living abroad comes to the UK every three months to care for her mum while the other siblings have an essential break.

Observe carefully how your parents are really functioning. No one ever wants to admit to failing faculties. Do not believe what is said because it is convenient or lets you dodge your duty.

OPTIONS

- Supporting parents in their own home
- Sheltered housing giving independence and support
- Sharing your home with infirm parents
- Finding accommodation in a residential home.

POINTS FOR CONSIDERATION

Option 1: may require considerable and increasing input to maintain safety and security. Moving to a more suitable house while still active is worth considering.

Option 2: is a physical and emotional upheaval for parents but gives security and safety.

Option 3: is demanding. Have you sufficient space? What of the effects on your children/marriage? How much daily input/support will be needed? Can you handle the reversal of roles? The increasing frailty? The constant watchfulness?

Option 4: research what is available. Try the *Which?* guide and the *Care Commission* website. Any decision depends on a range of factors requiring unemotional and informed discussion by all concerned.

Short-term memory loss

Be clear about the problems of dealing with short-term memory loss. Can you and the family acquire the necessary skills and the patience to cope with it?

The most effective method available at present for dealing with this condition is SPECAL (Specialised Early Care for Alzheimer's), which has three basic rules:

Don't ask questions

Never contradict

Learn to love their repetitiveness

Can you and your family adjust to all these factors?

Carers

Caring requires three facets of giving: emotional, mental and physical. It is all-encompassing. Be aware from the start that no one can give totally at all times. If the ability to help is destroyed, who will give the needed support?

However hard it sounds, it is essential to be organised and clear about the limits. The carer MUST have meaningful time away from the task to restore the ability to continue. If there are others, the care must be shared. If no others are involved then care must be sought or purchased.

Full nest syndrome

The return of the less than prodigal.

Just when you thought they were off the family payroll, back they come.

Money is the crux of the matter. If funds allowed then they would live elsewhere.

Mutual respect

Acknowledge from the beginning that this not the return of a child to the family home. The returnee is an adult. To live together harmoniously requires respect on both sides.

Parents must recognise that young adults have been used to considerable freedom. Moving back home can be very difficult for them. They have left behind their life of independence. They are rightly used to their personal affairs being just that. Give them privacy. Always knock on the door of bedrooms and wait for a response.

The returnee must recognise that parents have a lot less to gain from this set-up. Just when parents expected offspring to be independent, the costs increase, the daily rhythm is disrupted, freedom is curtailed and their quality of life diminished.

ACKNOWLEDGE THEIR ADULTHOOD

1. Beware of one partner letting things drift or acting as chauffeur, cook, etc., while operating a branch of the bank of Mum and Dad with 0% interest loans.
2. Never let your son or daughter live at home totally free. Arrange some form of payment and stick rigorously to it. Not doing so creates possible disagreements between parents and resentment.
3. Make the returnee take responsibility for her or his own actions. Don't allow flouting of the agreed rules. We are talking adults here. Adults who are going to hold down a job, budget a salary and run a household by themselves.
4. This is the last part of that parenting role that started in the neonatal unit. You have given all these years of care: are you going to fall at the last fence? Do not leave the job unfinished.

Never forget that to spoil has two meanings – to indulge and to do harm.

Communicate and cooperate

Hang on to your sanity, your marriage and your offspring's affection and respect by making clear the foundations of this new relationship from the beginning.

- *Keep the relationship functioning.* Address issues up front as they arise.
- *Establish boundaries.* Treat your offspring like any other adult. Independence mutually respected.
- *Rules must be set.* Negotiate reasonable rules for adults with both sides contributing.
- *Constructive family discussions.* Listen, discuss and negotiate an agreement. Review after 2–3 months.
- *Expect your rules to be respected.* No longer a child but a young adult. Be flexible on the ODD occasion.

Take time out

Family life is demanding so both parties need a break from each other on a daily basis as well as weekends away. Beware of staying up late just to have the house to yourself. This can lead to poor sleep patterns and short tempers.

Sanity sometimes needs intensive restoration: parents relaxing, offspring with friends. It is hard for the returnee to make the transition back into family life. He or she needs a life outside the home.

Communicate, communicate, communicate

This is the most important element.

If you do not talk openly to each other, how will you each know what is bothering you? How can you find a way forward, let alone a good compromise or even a solution? Both sides must talk about their concerns.

This relationship is not a one-way street but a two-way process.

Grandparenting

Being a grandparent offers you more roles than any theatre company, but some last only a few minutes. Much of the richness of your grandchildren's growing up will depend on how you play your role. It is easier to establish a really close bond with your grandchildren if you are part of their lives from the beginning. Create a special relationship with your grandchildren.

Grandparents need to be:

- **good listeners**
- **childminders**
- **peacemakers**
- **arbitrators**
- **agony aunts (and uncles)**
- **craft experts**
- **diplomats**
- **keepers of secrets**
- **but never, ever troublemakers.**

You too have a life to lead and the more fulfilling your life is the more you have to give your grandchildren. Organise your life so you can create and continue that special relationship. Which grandparent does not want to be a source of information and also to surprise their grandchildren by the unexpected other sides to their lives?

RULES FOR GRANDPARENTS

1. Make all the visits of grandchildren times of enjoyment.
2. Help them to see that there are different behaviours or rules for different places.
3. Introduce the idea that there are grandparent's rules in your house and garden.
4. Rules can be about fun too, and part of the pleasure of their visit.

Little ones: dealing with dangers

All small children need to explore the world around them. This means they will do things that are potentially dangerous. Just to say *stop* or *don't do that* does not tell the child that running in the road is seriously different from turning the yoghurt pot upside down.

Handle this by facing the children, holding their hands and, looking into their eyes, quietly, calmly and firmly telling them that they must not do ... because it could mean that they could be badly hurt and you want them to be safe and well. Your seriousness will mark out those danger areas for the children.

OLDER GRANDCHILDREN

- Learn to share the interests of your grandchildren.
- Information and knowledge between you should not be a one-way street.
- Take advantage of the brain stimulation from being part of their incredibly different world.

NOW FOR THE PARENTS

- Do not imply superiority about your rules against their parents' rules.
- Stress your rules are just different ones for a different place.
- Support the parents. Never undermine the parents openly or implicitly.
- Recognise that your grandchild's world is vastly different from that of your own child.
- Keep your opinions and beliefs to yourself until the parents ask for advice.
- Do not make public any areas of disagreement with the parents.
- Put Trappist monks to shame by the quality of your understanding silence.

Remember that you only brought up 50% of the parents and even that was not perfect!

AND THE OTHER GRANDPARENTS

- Under no circumstances criticise or openly disagree with the other grandparents.
- Do not express negative thoughts even to your own child about the other grandparents. That is unfair pressure and puts a strain on loyalty. Trappist rules apply, OK?
- Finally never, ever enter into a giving competition with presents. If the other grandma gives a bigger, better, shinier present than yours, so what? Does baby notice?

Change or departure of a parent

It takes love to work hard at being truthful or to omit to tell all. Above all you must have an eye to the future.

1. Keep a tight rein on what you say – they might just get back together! Your offspring and partner have to handle the break-up without your interference. After all they started the relationship, lived it and have broken it.
2. This is the time when your grandchildren need you most. You are the only unchanging part of the child's world, the stable person in the turbulence that has hit them.
3. Use one principle as a guide. Put your grandchild's needs in the central position. Use that as a measure of your actions. Such even-handedness will bring flak from both sides. Stating what you are doing and why might bring at least some grudging acknowledgement of the vital care you are giving.

ACCEPTING A NEW PARTNER

1. Do not endlessly go over what or who caused the break-up. You cannot change the actions of others. For you there is the loss of a son- or daughter-in-law who was part of your family.

2. Keep contacts open. The departing partner should still play a part in your grandchild's life so do not have a no-go area between you and the child. Try to be a bridge-builder. Accept the situation, put a lid on your sense of betrayal while you are with your grandchild. Remember who is in the centre, whose needs are greatest.

3. Accept the new partner, it is your child's choice. Welcome the new partner with as much warmth as you can for your grandchildren's sake. Your grandchildren need that. It is the reality of their lives. Keep their lives as stress-free as far as it is in your power, which may be greater than you think.

The best rule I have heard for grandparents in all circumstances is:

> **Stay calm, stay collected and stay out of it.**

Grief

The first reactions to the death of a partner or parent are often delayed because of having to make so many practical and necessary decisions and the need to respond to others who also care deeply.

When this time has passed, the reality can appear bleak, that these empty days will stretch to the end of life.

The fact of death does last forever and the relationship does too – in a different form. It will take time but eventually grief becomes more manageable if you let it. You will come to feel warmth and gratitude for the times that were shared together.

Holding on only to the sadness of your loss or to the anger at being left to cope alone diminishes the quality of the relationship you shared. It is not love. It is to reduce the person you claim to have loved to someone who has assisted you in your life – not someone who shared your life and enriched it.

Keeping going

When a much-loved person dies you think you will never really live again. There is no blueprint for surviving such a death. We can only get through by clutching onto some kind of support.

These guidelines have been found helpful:

- **One day at a time: plan just to get through the day. Do the little tasks that need to be done.**
- **Live in the present: don't look back, don't look forward. Live in the here and now.**
- **Recognise the anger: don't suppress the rage you feel. Take it out in physical action.**
- **Get back to a pattern: routine and distractions give shape and purpose to the day.**
- **Separate things out: don't make topics taboo. They are part of the daily life you need.**
- **Accept invitations: make yourself go out to meet others. Do not become a tragic person.**
- **Look after yourself: keep your self-respect. Don't let your appearance or your nutrition go.**
- **Have short-term manageable goals: write down one per day. Check in the evening.**

We have to make ourselves care about ourselves.

Sometimes we can do this by thinking of what our partner would have wanted us to do. How would he or she have expected us to restructure our day? How should we cope with returning to an empty house, an empty bed, a table set for one?

Everyone deals with grief in a different way.

No way is straightforward. Each has to find his or her own way through. Expect some days to be better or worse than others. We can be ambushed by grief – irrationally and irregularly. Expect this. We catch a glimpse of someone and, for a fleeting moment, our hearts leap because we think it is the one we love. We hear a joke and turn to share it but there's no one. These are the times that are so difficult. They can be in public places – shops or cafés or on the bus – and the need to appear in control adds to the pain that threatens to overwhelm.

No matter how well we make sense of our new life there will always be times of unhappiness.

Keep busy so that you don't go into the depths of unhappiness. Everyone has had unhappy times and come out of them. Have the confidence to believe that you will repeat what you have achieved previously.

Think of how to deal with your unhappiness, learn to balance it. Do not allow yourself to be dragged under by its weight: that is irresponsible and self-defeating.

> **The secret of carrying any burden is not to focus on its weight alone but on how to carry the weight.**

New partnership

Time may come when you find a companion or friend you value greatly.

Do not feel guilt at having had the good fortune to find someone you wish to be with. Would your partner have wanted you to pass up the possibility of happiness?

First a word of warning: be ruthlessly honest.

Ask yourself: is this the outcome of a search to fill a gap?

How much success can there be in a relationship where one is seeking only to satisfy what he or she needs? That is not a relationship; that is selfish abuse of another person. Such a person, often male, is a SANDY, someone *Seeking a Nurse or Domestic*. Ladies, you have been warned. Avoid SANDYs like the plague.

There is a difference between being open to the possibility of a new partner and looking for a new partner on the rebound from the pain of loss. It is true that those who have been happily married are more likely to marry again. Wanting to move on positively with life is not to betray your partner or your shared past. It is adaptation to reality. There is no going back: that is why the present is so important.

Finding a new partner in life

This is a stressful and hazardous undertaking at any stage in life but especially so at a later stage. The hazards and rewards are different.

What is valued are the very qualities ignored by youthful passion: the quieter joy of friendship and of shared interests and values. These increase the wonder of finding new love and of being loved anew.

Dating is totally transformed. Be wary of internet dating and newspaper lonely hearts columns. Where there is no background information fraudsters are harder to detect. Nevertheless many happy and lasting relationships began on the internet. Another way to make new contacts is through activity groups, supper clubs, etc. Expand your interests and your social life at the same time!

Do not rush into making any new relationship too fixed too early. Enjoy the gradual adjustment to each other's way of life and responsibilities. Love me, love my baggage may well have to be the mantra.

Returning to work

The reasons people return to work vary. The need to boost pensions may force re-entry into paid work. For others it is the desire to continue to do a job they enjoy. Some seize this chance to take risks by trying out new areas or hopeful dreams. The 50+ agers are one of the fastest-growing groups for start-up businesses.

Irrespective of the reason, resist the feeling to find work straight away.

TO MAKE SURE OF MAKING THE RIGHT MOVE, CONSIDER:

- **Type of work: previous area of work? New area? Current skills in new area?**
- **Length of work: full or part time? Flexitime? Jobshare?**

- Amount of responsibility: how much gives job satisfaction without stress?
- Skills needed: upgrade/expand current skills? Acquire new skills? Computer literacy?

> The only constant thing in life is change.

Financial reasons

Even with a pressing need to earn money, examine options thoroughly. Take time to think.

- Review your budget, calculate the cost of working, i.e. cost of travel, clothing, etc.
- Consider if a full-time or part-time job is needed. Be flexible, part-time may become full-time.
- What kind of activities/work do you want to do?
- Do you want to return to your previous work or to a new area?

Move when you have a clear sense of what you want.

- *Improve your employability.* Update computer skills to show preparation for new work.
- *Expand/improve skills through voluntary work.*
- *Rethink your CV.* Demonstrate how your skills and experience are relevant to the post. Indicate ability to develop new skills, to work in new areas. Use a modern layout with contact details, work profile, etc. Don't rest on past, possibly irrelevant glories, write more than two pages or give references.
- *Stick to a job search schedule.* Use the internet, job centres, newspapers, old contacts. Seek out 50+ employment

agencies. Contact firms with a policy of employment of mature workers e.g. B&Q, Asda.

- *Do not despise routine jobs.* Bar/till/shop work require the skills to be efficient, numerate, able to use your initiative, be part of a team and have customer-handling skills
- *Do not underrate your own abilities.* B&Q have shown how employing retired skilled tradesmen as shop assistants with real knowledge has boosted their image and profits.
- *Do not be ashamed of rejection.*
- *Do not neglect your social life.*

Continuing work

Be honest about your motivation to return to the world of work.

The most positive reason to continue working is that you have the energy, ability and commitment to contribute constructively. If later you organise a staged reduction of hours then you have the ideal preparation for transition to non-working life.

If, on the other hand, you confuse having a job or a career with having a life or continue working because you feel the loss of status or lack a challenge or purpose in life then there are problems. At some time the situation of life without work must be faced.

Use the return to work to plan a constructive retirement. Your knowledge and skills could be used to mentor others through commercial or charity networks. Consider also the possibility of working with VSO to create infrastructure in other countries. At least 28% of VSO volunteers are aged 50 or over. What a benefit your skills would be to another country!

Hopeful dreams

The greatest sadness in life is not to take the adventure. Now may be the time to do just that.

Start by developing your ideas and assessing the market. Test your idea by writing a business plan. Address issues of finance, location, starting costs, survival strategy, competition and publicity.

At this point contact organisations such as PRIME for constructive discussion and guidance. National and regional government schemes also exist. Running your own business can be lonely, so explore the benefits of having a knowledgeable mentor to give support and be a sounding board.

> **'Do the job you love and you'll never work a day in your life.'**
>
> —*Chinese proverb*

Life outwith the firm

The world of work is no preparation for the world outside. Satisfaction does not always figure highly let alone frequently in a number of jobs.

The joy of no longer working is the freedom to do what you want – so where to start? What to choose? How to make the best choices? Don't commit yourself too early; look around at the range of possibilities.

Exploration

List the things you enjoy doing and imagine doing these activities more often.

Would golf every day become more or less enjoyable than twice per week plus the monthly medal? Would the repetition of these activities expand your life into new areas, stimulate you, widen your social circle?

Now list all the things that you'd love to do, have ever thought of doing, wondered about trying once for the experience. Add to the list over a week.

Look at the list and highlight anything that is totally impossible. NASA will only let you on board if you have millions of pounds. Look again at the impossible and challenge yourself to find some way of reaching close to that activity or interest.

Leaving those special areas aside, divide your list into:

◾ **What you would do alone**
◾ **What you would do with one other**
◾ **What you would do in a group**
◾ **What you have always wanted to do.**

There may be limitations on your choices:

◾ *Legal barriers* – **no way round those.**
◾ *Physical limitations* – **you can get fitter. Look at less demanding forms of your choice. You do not have always to choose the most difficult. This is meant to be pleasurable!**
◾ *Financial constraints* **are real except for the super-rich. There are always alternatives if you seek them out. You can't afford a yacht, so what about crewing? You want long holidays in the sun, go in the off-season, take those last-minute deals.**
◾ *Self-limitation* – **this may be the time to go down that path you always wanted to explore.**

Carpe diem

Do things so that you can get the absolute best out of every experience. Don't wait or put things off. Regrets are much more about the things that were not done rather than the things that were done.

> **If you have always wanted to go somewhere, try some activity, see someone,**
>
> **DO IT NOW.**

APPENDIX 1

The Age Revolution progress chart

CONGRATULATIONS – how well did you perform?

- Did you manage to give yourself many small rewards?
- Did your achievements meet up with your expectations?
- Did you encounter many barriers to your changing lifestyle?

Now is the time to find out! You need feedback and you need to be honest! Remember, this programme is all about YOU so the only person you're fooling (if you don't tell the truth) is YOU! Rate the following performance indicators on a scale of 1–5, from lowest to highest. Be realistic: don't expect to be Arnold Schwarzenegger or Meryl Streep!

Fitness

	At commencement of programme	Where you are after 21 days	Where you want to be
Strength			
Flexibility			
Balance			
Diet and nutrition			

Weight			
Adherence to Programme			
Stress level			
TOTAL			

This provides a maximum 35 points per column. Column 1 charts your beginning. Column 2 charts your progress after 21 days. It doesn't matter where you begin; what matters is where you end! There is no success or failure in this programme; it is purely a personal journey to improve YOUR lifestyle and quality of life. If you have improved your score after 21 days by 10% – which is a very modest improvement – you will look better, feel better and be significantly healthier. You will be on the path to recovery, which is the most important step. Remember, you are reversing changes which have been developing over many years *and it is never too late to move forward!*

APPENDIX 2

Natural remedies

STRESS IS OFTEN described as a 'silent' disease but it has many effects which are less than silent! As described earlier, stress can produce many adverse effects on the body, from heart disease to insomnia, indigestion or even premature ageing of the skin! Poor circulation, reduced immunity and muscle spasm are proven effects of stress. Drugs are never an effective solution to the problem of stress, as medication treats only the *symptoms*, not the underlying cause of the problem. Techniques to lower or relieve stress are most effective without the use of drugs. In this context, the following have been found to be particularly effective:

Techniques to promote a calming influence

Frankincense

- Olibanum or frankincense oil is distilled from the resin of small trees found in India and southern Arabia.

- It has been used for thousands of years as incense and burned in churches for this purpose. The reasons for this are twofold: it is a natural antiseptic and therefore cleanses the atmosphere where large numbers of people are gathered; frankincense also has a reputation for a calming effect on the nervous system. Traditionally it is used to aid meditation and prayer, so it is a good oil to pop on a burner if you are stressed.

- It also seems to have a capacity to slow and deepen breathing, which soon produces a feeling of calm (see Chapter 4), while at the same time increasing energy.
- Finally, as mentioned on page 267, frankincense is also an excellent oil to improve the tone and hydration of the skin.
- It can therefore be used in many ways: on a burner, blended in a bath oil for relaxation or added to a cream base to make a rejuvenating skin moisturiser.

Essential oils make wonderful natural air fresheners, fragrancing a room as well as setting a mood of relaxation.

FRANKINCENSE FACE CREAM

50 ml base cream
5 drops frankincense essential oil
2 drops lavender or rose essential oil
2 ml (half a teaspoon) wheatgerm oil
2 ml (half a teaspoon) rosehip seed oil

FRANKINCENSE AND LAVENDER BATH OIL

50 ml base bath oil
5 drops frankincense essential oil
10 drops lavender essential oil

BLEND FOR AROMASTONE OR BURNER FOR MEDITATION AND RELAXATION

To a tablespoon of water add:

3 drops frankincense essential oil
1 drop lavender essential oil
2 drops geranium essential oil

(If you have only massage oil at home, make the blend in this then add a teaspoon of full-fat milk to 10 ml of the blend to act as a dispersant.)

Insomnia

There are several herbs that are good for insomnia. Sometimes blending 4–5 herbs together makes for a much more enjoyable tea.

■ **Passiflora is a calming and mildly sedative herb that acts as a natural tranquilliser.**
■ **Camomile is used to promote sleep and can be an acquired taste so mixing it in a blend will help disguise this.**
■ **Rose petals have a balancing effect on the nervous system, being both calming and uplifting. Use the rose petals sparingly in your blend as they have a powerful fragrance.**
■ **Lemon balm is a tonic for the nervous system that also alleviates insomnia. Balm grows in abundance in gardens, like mint, and is delicious as a fresh tisane. Tisane is easy to prepare by the following method:**

1. Add 1 teaspoon lemon balm per cup of hot water.
2. Cover with a saucer to capture the herb's volatile oils.
3. Leave to infuse for 5 minutes.
4. Strain and serve immediately.

OTHER STRATEGIES

■ **Having a warm bath with 4–6 drops of lavender essential oil to raise body temperature and soothe the mind can do wonders for a restful sleep. However, lavender oil used in large quantities is stimulating so don't overdo it if you are very tired and think that adding more will help. Less is more!**

Massage

Never underestimate the relaxing effects of massage! This can be achieved anywhere without any special equipment: the stress relief is equally effective.

HAND MASSAGE

■ **Massaging the hands keeps the skin soft and supple and prevents ageing.**

■ Start by using your right hand to massage your left hand, and vice versa.

■ Using your thumb make gentle rolling movements up and down each finger and thumb. Keep the pressure quite light.

■ Next, massage the palm of your hand with your thumb, making sure the pressure is more intense.

■ Finally, gently clasp your hands together and give them a gentle massage. Stretch and relax.

FACIAL MASSAGE

■ Good blood flow and lymph drainage are essential for supple, radiant skin.

■ With your fingers, massage in small circles outward from the centre of the chin to the earlobe, concentrating on the jaw line.

■ Return fingers to the corners of your mouth, and massage up to the middle of the ear; then return fingers to nostrils and massage to the temples.

■ Glide fingers back to chin to start over again; finish by pressing the pressure points at your temples.

■ Repeat each three times if you can.

Circulation and immunity

Arnica

Arnica is a plant that grows in the mountains where it has long been used to treat people injuring themselves from falling. It may increase peripheral circulation and therefore may be beneficial in the treatment of rheumatic and neuralgic pain.

■ A 6 cc dosage is the smallest dose and is more suitable for someone who is frail and also can be repeated more frequently if required. A 30 cc dose can be used for more acute pain like after a fall.

■ Remedies can be repeated as and when required.

■ Arnica salve can be used before and after exercise.

ARNICA SALVE

1 teaspoon beeswax
70g cocoa butter
1 teaspoon coconut oil
1 tablespoon arnica-macerated oil
1 tablespoon comfrey-macerated oil
1 tablespoon olive oil
4 drops lavender essential oil
3 drops rosemary essential oil
3 drops ginger essential oil

1. Melt the beeswax, cocoa butter and coconut oil in a basin over a saucepan of hot water.
2. Add arnica, comfrey and olive oil.
3. Add essential oils and stir well.
4. Pour into a dark glass jar before the mixture begins to harden.

This salve is effective for up to 6 months.

Macerated oils

Gardeners will often have an abundance of comfrey (old-fashioned name 'bone knit') so you may want to harvest this to make your own comfrey-macerated oil. Comfrey oil is a cooling oil which is beneficial as rubbing oil for sprains, aching limbs, arthritis and rheumatism.

1. Pack a sealable jar tightly with finely chopped comfrey leaves.
2. Cover with a good-quality vegetable oil. It is important that the plant material is completely covered by the oil for both the full extraction and to exclude contamination.
3. Seal the jar and leave in complete sunshine for 2 weeks (such as on the kitchen windowsill).

4. Strain and repeat with fresh plant material. Leave for another 2 weeks, shaking daily.
5. Strain, pour into a dark glass bottle and label.

The oil is effective for up to 12 months.

Ginger

Most of us are familiar with the warming 'comfort foods' that seem most appropriate during the winter months. Some foodstuffs such as ginger and garlic act as positive guards to our health. You can use more of them in your diet or introduce them in a number of other ways.

- The properties of ginger are stimulating and warming, and also a boost to the immune system.
- Ginger is an effective anti-emetic.
- In traditional Chinese households they believe that using ginger at the beginning of the winter will help to boost immunity, so that you are less likely to become ill as you move into the cold season.
- Ginger can be used in a wide variety of ways. You can use fresh or powdered ginger in food and drinks.
- Juicing is an excellent way to increase your intake of ginger; add a thumb-size piece of ginger to carrot, apple and celery for a good cleansing juice or substitute beetroot for the celery.
- Ginger salve massage has been used in the feet to stimulate circulation and has a general warming effect.

WARMING GINGER SALVE

20 g beeswax
15 drops ginger essential oil
10 drops rosemary essential oil
5 drops lavender essential oil
5 ml arnica-macerated oil

1. Heat the beeswax in a bowl set over a saucepan of boiling water.
2. Remove from heat and mix in all other ingredients.
3. Pour into a sterilised glass jar and allow to set.
4. Keeps for up to 6 months.

Prickly ash

The bark of the prickly ash tree, a native of North America, is a circulatory stimulant. It is said to stimulate the lymphatic system and therefore encourage the elimination of toxins, many of which are removed by lymphatics.

- Although it may seem strange for a therapeutic agent to originate in tree bark, you should remember that the acetylsalicylic acid in aspirin originates from the bark of the willow tree!
- Prickly ash has been attributed with antimicrobial qualities and as a pain-relieving agent – possibly as a similar mechanism to aspirin.
- In this context it has been used as a remedy for cramp when walking or swimming.
- Prickly ash is best taken in tincture form. It tastes slightly 'woody', but adding a little fruit juice will mask this.

Slippery elm

Acid reflux can be both painful and unpleasant and occurs more frequently as we age and our digestive system is not quite as efficient.

Slippery elm is one of nature's most soothing remedies for inflammation or ulceration anywhere along the digestive tract.

- It is nutritious and demulcent.
- It is postulated to protect the gastric mucosa from the erosive effects of too much acid.

- In a similar way, slippery elm powder can protect the oesophageal mucosa and relieves the pain of indigestion, giving lasting protection against acid reflux.
- It has been effectively applied before a journey to allay travel sickness.
- Slippery elm powder can be mixed with a little water or added to a mug of recently boiled water. It is relatively tasteless so can be mixed with a little cinnamon powder to make a pleasant drink.

Regenerative remedies for the skin

As the skin ages it loses elasticity and its ability to retain moisture, and fine lines and wrinkles appear. The emphasis on good skin care is on nourishing and moisturising to reduce the effects of the ageing process.

- Regenerative herbs for mature skin include rose and calendula (marigold). The number one essential oil is frankincense but rose, lavender and neroli are also beneficial.
- As we age the number of elastin fibres begins to decline rapidly, and collagen fibres become twisted and matted causing wrinkles and lines. However, there are measures that can be taken to minimise the damage and reverse some of the temporary damage.

Effective measures include the following:

- Avoiding the harmful effects of the sun and using a sunscreen.
- Free radical activity can be reduced by the use of antioxidants. Although free radical activity is most detrimental to our internal health (as explained in Chapter 2), the damage from free radical activity is most obvious externally on the skin. The most effective antioxidant for the skin is Vitamin E and so it's good to include wheatgerm oil, which is the richest source of Vitamin E, in your face cream.

■ Rosehip seed oil (*Rosa Mosqueta*), which is high in vitamin C, has a reputation for reducing wrinkles or sun-damaged skin. It is ideal to blend with other base oils or creams and can be used alone as an occasional night-time facial treatment.

■ Of course, one must not underestimate the importance of *internal* antioxidants in the diet in slowing the effects of ageing as described in Chapter 2. Your diet has a greater effect than external oils in preventing the development of wrinkles. Important antioxidants include vitamins A, C and E, plus selenium and zinc, which are found in fresh fruit and vegetables.

■ And never underestimate the importance of fresh air and exercise.

Index